"This is a fantastic read! Utterly enjoyable, arrestingly honest — a great companion to anyone on the yogi's path. With incredible insight and humor, Brian has captured the story of our generation of seekers."
— Rolf Gates, author of *Meditations from the Mat*

"Reading Brian's book and seeing how much he has benefited physically and mentally from his yoga practice not only makes for great reading but will inspire people to begin their own journeys. Great job, Brian!"
— Bryan Kest, creator of Power Yoga

"Brian Leaf's book is hilarious, inspiring, and poignant — and often all three on the same page! I love the eight Keys to Happiness — a perfect recipe for peace and freedom!"
— Amy Ippoliti, yoga instructor and creator of 90 Minutes to Change the World

"I am touched by Brian's sincere and steady desire to know what is true and to be in alignment with life."
— Jonathan Foust, senior teacher at and former president of the Kripalu Center for Yoga and Health

"In this delightful memoir, Brian Leaf recounts his early adventures as an over-educated, itinerant yogi. He writes in an utterly winning voice — by turns as neurotic as Woody Allen, as irreverent as Huck Finn, and as serious as Jack Kerouac. It's a fun romp — and much, much more. Leaf wisely structures his narrative around many of the most important pillars of yoga philosophy and practice — and he metes them out in doses that are easy to swallow. Seekers of all stripes will be happy to have this book: it's a great read and a quintessentially American doorway into the perennial philosophy of yoga."
— Stephen Cope, director of the Kripalu Institute for Extraordinary Living and author of *Yoga and the Quest for the True Self*

"From its first hilariously humiliating image to its closing words of grace, Brian Leaf's memoir is an unfolding miracle. Don't be fooled. This is not for yogis only but a quest for self-knowledge that transcends its title. Leaf brings to his search piercing honesty, a willingness to share the embarrassments of being human, a survivor's sense of humor, and an opening and loving heart. Join him in seeking happiness, health, and love with practical tips that bring personal change within reach of us all." — Rebecca Pepper Sinkler, former editor of *The New York Times Book Review*

"Reading this book was like a flashback to my own formative years of seeking spiritual guidance. Along with all the inspirations always come the heartbreaks and disillusionments. Brian's writing is funny and accessible and clearly reflects his personality and life experience. Check it out!"

— Noah Levine, author of *Dharma Punx*

"This awesome book made me laugh out loud. I kept thinking, it's high time that a man told his *Eat, Pray, Love* story. That said, as a woman, I too could relate to Brian's journey. His writing is hilarious and insightful, and it brought back my own memories of the good, the bad, and the humorous along the road to awakening consciousness. Funny, real, and heartwarming." — Desirée Rumbaugh, yoga teacher and creator of the *Yoga to the Rescue* DVD series

"Brian Leaf is like the Bill Cosby of yoga — recounting common emotions and situations on a yogi's path in a way that makes you laugh with acknowledgment. His story is so graphic, I felt like I was practically holding his hand! This book is a great reminder of why everyone needs a little yoga — a true dose of physical, emotional, and mental medicine." — Kathryn Budig, yoga teacher and author of *The Women's Health Big Book of Yoga*

"Brian Leaf's charming and engaging account of his yogic journey is sure to strike a chord with readers who are embarking on their own adventures toward health and self-discovery."

— Leslie Kaminoff, yoga teacher and author of *Yoga Anatomy*

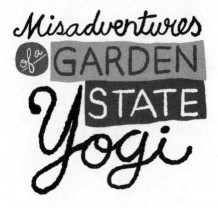

Misadventures of a Garden State Yogi

My Humble Quest to Heal My Colitis, Calm My ADD, and Find the Key to Happiness

Brian Leaf

New World Library
Novato, California

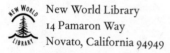

New World Library
14 Pamaron Way
Novato, California 94949

Text design by Tona Pearce Myers

Library of Congress Cataloging-in-Publication Data
Leaf, Brian.
 Misadventures of a Garden State yogi : my humble quest to heal my colitis, calm my ADD, and find the key to happiness / Brian Leaf.
    p.   cm.
Includes bibliographical references and index.
ISBN 978-1-60868-136-5 (pbk. : alk. paper)
 1. Leaf, Brian. 2. Yoga—Health aspects. I. Title.
RM727.Y64L43 2012
613.7'046—dc23   2012021383

First printing, October 2012
ISBN 978-1-60868-136-5
Printed in the USA on 100% postconsumer-waste recycled paper

 New World Library is proud to be a Gold Certified Environmentally Responsible Publisher. Publisher certification awarded by Green Press Initiative. www.greenpressinitiative.org

10 9 8 7 6 5 4 3 2 1

To Swami Kripalu

You have no idea how your life is gonna improve
as a result of this. Food tastes better.
The air seems fresher. You'll have more energy
and self-confidence than you ever dreamed of.

— JERRY SEINFELD, *Seinfeld*, "The Shower Head," 1996

Contents

Preface

The Rolling Incident

There's surely an uneven power dynamic between one person sitting naked on the toilet and the other hovering above in a dark suit. This is especially and egregiously true if the person sitting is pushing to no avail.

Such was the case as I sat naked in Dr. Brenner's special post-colonoscopy bathroom. He wanted to speak with me about the results and was already late for his next appointment, so he walked on in and started to chat while I was on the potty. At the end of our talk, he offhandedly said, "If you're having trouble relieving the gas, we can roll you."

I was game for anything.

So two nurses laid me out on the crinkly paper of an examining table and rolled me back and forth. Their goal was to move things around and let the gas out.

This worked marvelously, and I was both enormously relieved and atrociously humiliated — until I recognized one of the nurses as the mother of a girl I had a huge crush on in school, and then I was only atrociously humiliated.

Thankfully, though, a dedicated yoga practice, which has included wearing winter gloves and punching a mattress as I shout

Sanskrit chants, has cured me of colitis and spared me future humiliations. But I'm getting ahead of myself.

It all started when I was sixteen years old, during the fall of my senior year of high school. I remember being slumped on the couch, watching *Laverne & Shirley* reruns. Shirley was vacuuming, and I thought to myself, "How does she have the energy to do that? It looks so exhausting."

I was in bad shape. But I had trouble telling anyone about my embarrassing symptoms, so it took a while for me to tell my family, and then a while for us to find the right doctor.

Eventually we found Dr. Brenner, a gastroenterologist, and he scheduled a battery of tests. At this point the true humiliation began. I was already lethargic and losing weight because my body was not digesting food properly — I weighed 142 pounds, which is not much at six-foot-two — and now I had to undergo colonoscopies. Colonoscopies are supposed to be reserved for seventy-two-year-old men and repeat alien abductees from North Dakota who expect this sort of violation. One time the doctor showed me how much rubber tubing had been involved in that particular day's probe: a full three feet.

As if the basics of a colonoscopy are not bad enough, during such an exam, when the fiber-optic tube is deep up in there, the doctor has to be able to see the wall of the colon, so he pumps in gas. One time I had trouble relieving the gas, and that's what led to the rolling incident.

After the tests, Dr. Brenner diagnosed me with ulcerative colitis.

I had colitis because I was a stressed-out kid — I was a straight-A student, the champion debater of New Jersey, and president of the Spanish Club.

Spanish Club might sound quaint, and it was. As president my one responsibility was to coordinate our monthly Spanish dinner. The dinner entailed, basically, getting together in the home ec room to heat up nachos, cook *arroz con pollo*, and convince Sra. Moran that there was no drinking age in the United Sates. But for some reason the mirth of all this was lost on me, and every month I was a wreck, like Adrian Monk planning a presidential state dinner.

After the diagnosis, Dr. Brenner started me on some meds. They took a while to kick in, but by the summer I was better. And the timing was excellent, because in the fall I was to attend Georgetown University.

After that first ten-month battle with colitis, I vowed never to take a healthy bowel movement for granted, and I'm proud to say that for twenty years I have succeeded valiantly in this department. Still today, in fact, I often find myself down on my hands and knees examining the evidence with the gratitude, wonder, and delight of *The Last Emperor*'s court physician.

During my first two years at Georgetown, I was blessedly colitis-free. But even so, I realized how deeply stressed I was, and that though I knew how to get As, I knew little about how to be comfortable, relaxed, and happy. I wanted desperately to feel more at ease. I wanted to feel more loving and more free-spirited. So I started doing experiments to learn how to live.

In one experiment I decided to follow my urges and whims exclusively. I imagined that if I studied when I felt like studying, I'd be most productive at those times, and that if I felt like hanging out with friends or working out, I should do those things then, when my intention was strongest.

I think there's really something to this. And I see now that this has always been my foundational practice: trusting in the intelligence of true desire, authentic intuition, and flowing energy. This practice has influenced my biggest decisions, has informed my professional life, and eventually led me to Kripalu yoga.

But unfortunately, that particular experiment failed...quite miserably. After three weeks, I awoke one morning (severely behind on reading and writing for my classes), wearing the same clothes that I had been in for several days, with vomit on my shirt where a woman had puked on me the night before, and with a sprained ankle from earlier that same night when she and I had jumped a fence so we could hook up on the fifty-yard line of the Georgetown football field.

I needed some discipline and some honing of my intuition before I could completely release to the flow.

For the decade following that project, I explored, I traveled, I trained, and I experimented. I searched for ways to feel comfortable and happy. I consulted psychics, scientists, yogis, swamis, Ayurvedic physicians, life coaches, and even (*accidentally, I assure you*) a prostitute. I tried meditation, herbs, flower essences, psychotherapy, and shouting out my angst. I *almost* tried sesame oil enemas, walking on hot coals, and urine therapy (the daily practice of drinking one's own midstream morning urine).

And I learned a lot.

From yoga, I learned how to stand and how to breathe.

From yoga's sister science, Ayurveda, I learned how to eat, how to poop, and how to sleep.

From meditation and Kripalu yoga, I learned to awaken my feelings and my intuition.

And from Jerry Garcia, Misha the yogi, and a scary shaman named Genevieve, I learned to emote, to connect, and to love.

During this journey, I found eight Keys to Happiness, eight rules to live by for health and vitality. Eight principles, each powerful in its own right, but the first seven trumped by the final and eighth key.

And with these keys, I healed my colitis, calmed my ADD, ignited my intuition, and opened my heart. And, luckily for me, without a single sesame oil enema, without walking on hot coals, and without sipping even one Dixie cup of my own morning urine, I learned how to feel more comfortable, more authentic, more relaxed, and happier.

But, again, I'm getting ahead of myself. So let's take it back two decades to begin our tale in the time of Bill Clinton; the Beastie Boys; *Beverly Hills, 90210*; and the United Colors of Benetton...

THE EIGHT KEYS TO HAPPINESS

Do yoga. And if you already do yoga, do *more* yoga.

Follow your heart.

Cultivate and follow your intuition.

Apply at least three pieces of Ayurvedic wisdom
to your daily schedule.

Meditate.

Connect with your heart, and interact with others
from that place.

Speak and act from your true self.

Become most real.

BOOK ONE

Turning On

Chapter 1

Moooola Bannnda

I didn't plan on getting so involved with yoga; I sort of stumbled into it.

When I was a senior in high school, my brother, Larry, was attending the University of Virginia. The school is very large, so it can offer all sorts of fun electives, and there are enough students to fill even the most peculiar classes. During his first semester, Larry took kung fu and riflery, and in the second semester he took skeet shooting and a class that helped train him to run a marathon. After the marathon, Larry's nipples were so chafed from rubbing against his sweaty shirt that he had to wear a Band-Aid on each side for a week.

Larry's kung fu and riflery classes had us joking that he was covertly training for the CIA, but after the Band-Aids, as well as a miniature golf elective, we dropped the joke. We couldn't see James Bond needing Band-Aids to protect nipple boo-boos.

So at the end of my senior year of high school, sitting on my toy soldier–themed comforter, I was preregistering for my Georgetown classes, and I wanted to round out my humanities and business courses with something similar to what Larry had taken at UVA. Georgetown is a smaller school, so fewer courses are offered. I was choosing between jazz dance, squash, step aerobics, and yoga. I selected yoga as the most exotic choice.

Five months later, on day one of yoga class, I'm sitting on a long bench outside a classroom in Georgetown's Yates athletic building waiting for the teacher to show up. This is 1989, so as you visualize this scene, incorporate lots of very tight spandex, neon sweatbands, leg warmers, and feathered hair. It will also help if you include a few Members Only jackets and a pair of acid-washed jeans, and perhaps hum Bon Jovi's "I'll Be There for You" or Madonna's "Like a Prayer" as a quiet sound track.

I'm waiting on the bench as woman after woman shows up. We've got freshmen, sophomores, juniors, and seniors, and grad students, and they're *all* women. No other men. At all. I am brand-new to yoga, so I have no idea what's going on. I am seventeen years old and surrounded by thirty-one women, all wearing tight spandex. You'd think I'd feel great about this ratio, but, frankly, I'm terrified. I wonder if I am mistakenly sitting outside a woman's gathering of some sort. Perhaps "Menstruation and You" or "A Woman's Guide to Dating at Georgetown," or, worst-case scenario, "Aquatic Jazzercise."

Why were there no other men on the bench outside that yoga class? Answer: this was 1989, before many guys did yoga. Men can now hug and cry and do yoga and drink white wine and wear an apron and cook free-range chicken picatta. But in 1989 we were pretty much hemmed in between Al Bundy and Magnum P.I. — limited to watching televised sports, eating large pieces of meat, and drinking cheap beer stored in a small fridge next to the couch.

Even with the skewed demographic on the wooden benches,

before long I knew I was indeed in the right place, waiting for a yoga class, because soon the yoga teacher showed up. And he was unmistakably the yoga teacher. Either that, or he was from the drama department and had come straight from Georgetown's production of *The Ten Commandments*.*

Oskar even looked Indian to me (though I later found out that he was Peruvian). He had a big Alan-from-*The-Hangover* beard, his clothes were all white, and he was wearing leather sandals. These days, stockbrokers, accountants, and off-duty construction workers proudly wear Birkenstocks, but back then leather sandals on a man sent a very specific message, a message like, "This man and these feet are free, as God made them. And this man thinks about foot health. And he likes to close his eyes and smile placidly as he breathes deeply in the fresh air. And he does not own a TV and certainly has not seen Michael Jordan's Nike commercials."

☙

Right before that first yoga class I had been at the Georgetown University debate team building. I had not been recruited to Georgetown for debate, and I had not even contacted the coach; I was planning to be a walk-on to the team. But first I showed up anonymously to check it out. Really, I think I just wanted to make a dramatic entrance when I finally announced to the coach and to the team my true identity as debate royalty (being debate champ of New Jersey is like being ice-dancing champ of Russia).

---

* There was no other explanation as to why a man at Georgetown would not be wearing either the 1980s-era exercise attire as described above or the requisite Georgetown men's unofficial uniform of khaki pants, bucks, baseball cap, and tucked-in white, pink, or blue button-down shirt.

But, during my anonymous tour of the place, I was appalled. One of the debaters, who resembled Draco Malfoy in every way, showed me around and informed me, "No one *walks* onto the *Georgetown* debate team." Then I sat with Coach Snape and learned that debate team at Georgetown was a full-time gig and that the people I met, including Severus and Draco, would be my new family.

Here's a transcript of my thoughts as I left the meeting to rush off to my first yoga class:

"I was debate champ of New Jersey, for sobbing out loud. I have to join."

"But I don't want to."

"You have to. There are expectations. And you're very good at it."

Enter Oskar in his sandals, beard, and all whites.

Yoga class began with the prayer of St. Francis, "Lord, make me an instrument of your peace. Where there is hatred, let me sow love" and ended with "Let there be peace on Earth. Let peace begin with me. Let there be peace on Earth, the peace that was meant to be."

I imagine that these blessings were part of Georgetown's compromise with Oskar in allowing him to teach yoga at a Jesuit school. For most of my yoga classmates, these prayers probably evoked thoughts of Easter bonnets and dusty church pews. But I had grown up Jewish and had never heard them before (I imagined they were straight from the Bhagavad Gita), so I heard them with fresh ears, and they, along with the yoga warm-ups, poses, and guided relaxation, awoke something in me. After forty minutes of breathing deeply and bending myself in all manner of new ways, I felt more relaxed and at ease than I could remember.

I felt like I was in exactly the right place. I had been faking it as a debater. Debate was work, and while I enjoyed the praise I received after winning, I had never enjoyed the actual debating. I don't even like to argue.

Oskar's yoga class touched the right chord and made my soul sing. I had signed up for yoga on a lark, but even in that first class, I knew what I had found.

Lying in relaxation pose at the end of class, I realized:

"This feels good."

"I'm going to be doing this a lot."

"Wow, I am not going to join the debate team."

This was a telling moment of insight that describes how I have attempted to make decisions ever since. I seek not to decide but to relax and calm my mind enough to simply realize and feel the correct path before me. I know that this places me dangerously close to the decision-making behavior of an invertebrate, or even of George W. Bush, but I will clear that up later on.

I became a yoga zealot pretty quickly. I loved feeling, for the first time, the muscles between my ribs as I stretched in *setu bandhasana* (bridge pose). I loved the prayers — this was the first time I had taken seriously a charge to effect world peace — and I loved the relaxation. Oskar's deep, euphonic voice soothed every muscle in my body, and when he said "relaaaax," I melted.

One day after class I told Oskar about my colitis. He recommended that I practice "[insert *deep, relaxing voice*] moooola bannnda" sixty times a day. He explained, "Tense ouup and then relaaaax your anouuuse" thirty times every morning and thirty times every night.

Say again? Oskar had a pretty thick accent, and I was sure that I must have misheard him. He could not possibly have told me to tense and then relax my anus sixty times a day.

In fact, I doubt that I had ever, in my eighteen years, heard anyone speak about my anus at all before. Sure, I had heard the word used, but not in the context of my anus and certainly not by a bearded and sandaled yoga teacher dressed all in white.

Pursing my lips, squinting slightly, and bobbing my head like I was earnestly considering his wise counsel, I thanked him politely as I backed away. For days I shook my head and puzzled at what in the world he *possibly* could have said that sounded so much like *anus*.*

---

* Years later, in my studies of yoga, I learned of the *bandhas*, or "locks," as they translate into English, and sure enough there was *mula bandha*, a practice of lifting the muscles in the pelvic floor, from pubis to rectum, as in Kegel exercises. And *mula bandha*, the book instructed, could be used therapeutically for, among other things, ailments of the gastrointestinal tract. So it happened that Oskar was, of course, spot-on!

Chapter 2

Six-Packs

All life is an experiment.
The more experiments you make the better.

— RALPH WALDO EMERSON, journal, November 11, 1842

I wanted to practice and study yoga as much as possible, so I incorporated it into my Georgetown classes in every way that I could. For philosophy class, I wrote a paper entitled "Was Plato the Founder of Yoga?" (Unlike many modern philosophers, let's say, for example, Woody Allen, Plato believed that a sound mind requires a sound body, and in fact, the word *Plato* means "broad shoulders.") And for Catholic imagination class I wrote "Did Jesus Do Yoga?" (By the way, believe it or not, he did. Maybe. There is some pretty good evidence that sometime during his "lost years," between the ages of twelve and thirty, Jesus might just possibly have journeyed to India and Tibet and intensively studied yoga and Buddhism.)

Sophomore year of college I moved with a bunch of friends into a house way off campus. To avoid the extra round-trips to school, I took a semester off from Oskar's yoga at Yates and found a class right around the corner from my house. This class offered a differ-ent style of yoga, called Iyengar. Until then I had not imagined that there could be different schools of yoga. I thought, "Yoga is yoga, like basketball is basketball."*

But I learned that Oskar taught a type of Sivananda yoga. A Sivananda yoga class includes a bit of everything: chant, breathing exercises, meditation, poses, relaxation. And if Sivananda yoga is the five-course meal, or even the buffet table of yoga, then Iyengar yoga is the curmudgeonly dietician who demands that you sit up straight while you chew.

My Iyengar yoga class met in a junior high school gymnasium. We were supposed to bring a towel to practice on, but a towel offered little padding, and I usually forgot mine anyway, so I'd wind up practicing right on the hardwood floor. This was 1990, before the popularity of the now-ubiquitous "sticky mat" that you can purchase at Whole Foods, Target, and any gas station.† (Okay, maybe not the gas station, but I think they're headed there soon, along with the full line of Prana yoga wear.)

Beyond the superficial discomfort of elbows and knees on the cold gym floor and the resulting flashbacks of elementary school dodgeball humiliations, I enjoyed the class. I missed the relaxed flow of yoga postures and the overt spirituality of Oskar's yoga classes,

---

* By the way, don't let this cool basketball reference fool you into thinking I knew anything about basketball. I was an odd duck at Georgetown, caring nothing for the sport. The extent of my knowledge included knowing that Alonzo Mourning and Dikembe Mutombo (both at Georgetown at the time) were very tall. And I recall that Dikembe had an unbelievably deep voice.

† Sticky mats were invented, by the way, in the 1980s by Western yogi Angela Farmer from simple carpet padding, like the stuff under the rug in your den. And it was Sara Chambers of Hugger Mugger who took the nascent yoga mat industry to the next level in the 1990s by designing a mat of similar texture, made specifically for yoga. That's when the sticky mat that you now know and love was born and popularized. All rejoiced at this innovation, especially the tigers of India (whose skins were the choice mat for Indian yogis of yore).

but I appreciated the Iyengar teacher's detailed instructions for the proper alignment in each posture.

That year, I also began practicing a bit of yoga every day on my own, even when I went home to New Jersey on school breaks. (Though, in New Jersey, when someone goes into a room by himself to "meditate" and emerges thirty minutes later looking glassy-eyed and refreshed, there is all sorts of elbowing and winking, "Yes, he's been *meditating*, if you know what I mean, nudge, nudge, wink, wink.")

To connect with other yogis, I started subscribing to *Yoga Journal* magazine and visiting yoga centers in Washington, DC. I even sent away for a giant laminated poster of Dharma Mittra, demonstrating 908 postures. It's fair to say that if there had been a yoga chess set in pewter, I'd have had two. I was a full-scale yoga buff.

It was also that year that my colitis flared up again. My doctor had told me that colitis comes back at intervals and that everyone has their own period of return. It looked like mine was two years. I was devastated and flew home to New Jersey to see my doctor, get violated by three feet of rubber tubing, and start treatment.

After a *very* long weekend, I returned to Georgetown armed with a pharmacy bottle of sulfasalazine pills and several six-packs of Rowasa enemas. I think I can speak definitively for all nineteen-year-old boys when I say that amid the busy schedule of studying, partying, and attempting to meet women, I had no wish to steal away into a dorm bathroom and issue myself an enema. I was no fonder of colitis, however, and so I did it several times daily, feeling quite deflated and sullied each time.

Over the next three weeks, my symptoms persisted, even with the treatment. I began again to lose weight and become lethargic. Two years earlier Dr. Brenner had told me that when the symptoms returned they might be more difficult to control. He had even mentioned the possibility of surgery and a colostomy bag. I was sad and scared.

The doctor had also told me that the medicine would make me temporarily sterile, but that I could go off it later in life when I wanted to have children. Even at age nineteen, when I felt as close to having children as to retiring, this side effect disturbed me. Something that made me temporarily sterile seemed a pretty harsh substance to put into my body.

As fate would have it, though, I needed the meds for only a little longer, because the following week something unexpected and somewhat miraculous happened.

One evening in October 1990, I noticed that my symptoms were worse on days that I had skipped yoga. And I wondered, therefore, if doing more yoga would lessen the symptoms. For me, this was a giant leap. I had never heard of a mind-body connection. I had no clue that the choices I made could affect my health. I know that sounds crazy, but I was that ignorant.

Once I made the connection, I decided to medicate my condition with yoga. I self-medicated with four sun salutations, followed by ten minutes of deep relaxation, five times a day.

Taking these twenty-minute yoga breaks five times every day was a huge time investment. But it felt like the right thing to do.

I was a man on a mission. I was Rocky in *Rocky IV*.

And my effort proved worthwhile.

Because three days later my symptoms were gone.

GONE!

No losing weight and becoming lethargic. No medicine that made me sterile. No colostomy bag.

I was elated.

᪥

It actually makes perfect sense that yoga would help colitis. Sun salutations involve a repeated sequence of forward- and backward-bending yoga postures. These poses stretch, relax, and massage the muscles and organs in the abdomen and stimulate circulation and energy flow — all of which increases oxygen levels and improves cellular waste removal.

Furthermore, colitis is an ulcer in the colon, and like any ulcer it is affected by and possibly even caused by stress. Exercise, and especially gentle exercise paired with deep, relaxed breathing, triggers a parasympathetic nervous response (referred to as a "relaxation response") that helps relieve the stress. Many people, like me in 1990, spend all day in a sympathetic nervous state (a fight-or-flight stress response), and yoga literally resets the body's stress switch from stress response to relaxation response.

Yoga also helped me gain awareness of my body and my belly so that I could notice when I was tensing up and then release and relax those muscles. In addition, yoga taught me to stand straight rather than slouched over. I used to stand like Bull in *Night Court*. Perhaps I didn't want others to feel small, or maybe I was just trying to hear my girlfriend, who measured in at a grand total of four-foot-eleven.

Better posture is good for the organs. Picture your colon or liver working hard but being squished in an awkward position between your hipbone and ribs as you slouch over a computer. Now picture your organs resting freely in your body. Uncramped, they have better circulation and are better able do their jobs. Indeed, improving posture to uncramp the lungs is the first thing singers are taught: "If you want to project your voice you need bigger lungs, so stand up straight."

You can try this right now. Slouch and try to breathe a slow, deep breath. Then do the same thing while sitting up straight. In fact, a full, relaxed breath, impossible while slouched, actually triggers a relaxation response.

Ten minutes of deep relaxation five times a day would change anyone's life, whether or not he or she suffered from colitis. Imagine how relaxed and focused we'd all be, all that tiredness and irritability gone. I think we'd see the end of all war and hostility, a full-scale Age of Aquarius, if we all rested for ten minutes every three hours.

From a holistic health perspective, I'd say that my colitis was a condition of repressed angst pooling in my abdomen. In Western allopathic medicine we speak only metaphorically about emotion acting on our organs, and even then the quack police are readied for dispatch, but in the medicine of yoga, called Ayurveda, there is an actual language for this. Repressed anger affects the small intestine and the liver. Repressed anxiety affects the colon. Ayurveda literally states that disease happens when repressed or blocked energy pools and overflows into an incorrect channel. My ability to express and release angst was blocked, so the angst, with nowhere to go, pooled and pooled, and eventually, like acid, ate an ulcer into my colon wall.

Sun salutations massaged my muscles and organs, moved things around, broke up the blocks, and allowed some of the pooled energy to flow and release. This gave my colon wall a chance to heal itself, just as a cut on my finger would mend on its own. As the famous physician of integrative medicine Dr. Andrew Weil states, "Wounds heal by themselves....If we want to foster healing and promote health, we should...encourage the body's own, innate mechanisms of self repair."* Stretching, relaxing, resting, reducing my stress level, exercising, improving my circulation and energy flow, and straightening my posture were supporting this innate process in my body.

---

* *Family Guide to Natural Medicine: How to Stay Healthy the Natural Way* (New York: Reader's Digest, 1993), 8.

Chapter 3

Chicken Sandwiches

Yoga is the practice of tolerating the consequences
of being yourself.

— BHAGAVAD GITA

*M*y friend Paul and I had bonded over the chicken sandwiches
served in the dorm cafeteria on Tuesdays, and we always
made sure to be at lunch together on chicken-sandwich day. But
as I woke up to my body and how things affected it, I recognized
a cause-and-effect loop: on Tuesdays after I ate the chicken sand-
wich, I felt gross, as if oil was leaking out of my pores, as if there
was a vile, indigestible mass in my stomach. These were the kind of
processed chicken patties that look like breaded sponges with little
nooks and crannies of fat and the occasional chewy piece of carti-
lage that makes you look both ways before hunching over into your
napkin.

So finally, one Tuesday, I broke it to Paul that I wouldn't be
having the chicken that day. He was pretty upset. I didn't blame him;
this was our routine, a cornerstone of our fledgling friendship. Later
I broke it to him that I was giving up the chicken sandwiches per-
manently.

First I gave up the processed chicken patties. Then, I ate less
sugar, less fast food, and less processed junk. I was still a few years

15

away from eating brown rice, kale, and tempeh, but I was on the right track.

Giving up the chicken sandwiches was a turning point for me. It was a harbinger of many future pronouncements, seemingly odd quirks, and even embarrassing epiphanies that resulted from my yoga practice.

In 1994 I had to tell a landlord that I couldn't keep an office space because the "energy" wasn't right.

In 1999 I had to break it to Linda that we couldn't have sex in the mornings because it affected my morning yoga practice.

In 2000 I realized that I needed to learn how to feel and express anger, so in order to practice, I called everyone I had ever been angry at to tell them exactly how I felt.

And in 2002 I had to tell Millie that we couldn't cuddle at night as we fell asleep because I was practicing Reiki (a form of energy healing) on myself.

But back to college in 1993, when during senior year, like clockwork, my colitis flared up after two years of remission.

I noticed the symptoms early, and I took immediate action. Since my last bout of colitis, I had weaned myself down to practicing yoga twice and eventually once a day. So now, without pharmaceutical help, I again began my self-medicating treatment — four sun salutations followed by deep relaxation, five times a day.

Miraculously, like the last time, after only a few days, the symptoms disappeared. Again I was elated and grateful and ever more committed to yoga and holistic health.

I wanted to tell my doctor about all that was happening, but I had heard a story about a woman with breast cancer. She had dived headfirst into natural health, visiting alternative health practitioners and staying in spas, ashrams, and mountain retreats all over the world. She found something that worked for her, and the cancer disappeared. She shared the thrilling news with her doctor. He responded, "Impossible, there's no way that changing your diet and getting massages can have made the cancer disappear." She believed him because he was her doctor. She was devastated. The cancer returned, and within six months she was dead.

This story haunted me, and I was terrified to tell Dr. Brenner about my yoga cure. I believed in it. But did I believe in it strongly enough to hold resolute if he dismissed it?

I avoided him and canceled my checkups.

But, eventually, during a visit home, at the urging of my parents, I faced Dr. Brenner. I thought that in the best-case scenario he'd call me nuts, and in the worst-case scenario, well, who knows.

But instead, he nodded, "Yeah, I've heard that yoga can help colitis. There have even been a few studies."

Dr. Brenner looked me right in the eye, probably for the first time. We shared a moment. I thought he had joined me, was right there with me in my zealous commitment to yoga. Another convert, ready to swap out his scrubs for sweats. And truthfully, I think he was. I think he acknowledged the possibilities, even saw for a moment the potential to rise above society's addiction to pharmaceuticals, but then he shook his head slightly, as if waking from a daydream, made a sound like "Uunc," blinked a few times, and seemed to forget all about it. He jotted a few indecipherable notes in my folder and left the room. I never saw him again.

✍

This brings us, finally, to the first of our eight Keys to Happiness:

Do yoga. And if you already do yoga, do *more* yoga.

Yoga cured my friend Trish's chronic and debilitating back problems. Laigne, a coworker, had always suffered from having one leg a quarter inch shorter than the other. That threw off her hips, her spine, and her gait. She could barely run. Until she started doing yoga. Now she's strutting with ease. And, obviously, it changed my life.

So join me by doing some yoga. And if you're new to yoga, don't try only one class. Finding the right style of yoga is like dating. You might have to try various styles before you find the one for you. There's a spectrum of classes, from power vinyasa, if you like a vigorous workout, to gentle restorative, if you prefer something much cushier. So try at least three different yoga styles in your area. Look for yoga centers, or check bulletin boards at the library or health food store. You can also try a Google search for "yoga class [your town]."

In the meantime, while you're dating a few styles, you can also use appendix 1, which offers a simple yoga flow for you to practice right at home. You can record yourself reading the directions and then play them back as you practice, or if you can't say the word *buttocks* without giggling, you can download a recording of me guiding the practice at www.Misadventures-of-a-Yogi.com.

Chapter 4

Belly Down

Named must your fear be before banish it you can.

— JEDI MASTER YODA

*A*fter graduating from Georgetown, I moved into an apartment with my brother for one last year of living together before he got married (we had shared a room in my parents' house since I was one). We rented an apartment in Jersey City, New Jersey, across the Hudson River from Manhattan. From our window we could see the Statue of Liberty and all of lower Manhattan.

I took a job as a high school math teacher. I had started Georgetown four years earlier as a champion debater and future corporate attorney, but I graduated as a yogi math teacher. You already know about the debater-to-yogi transition that happened on day one of Oskar's yoga class. The other transition, from lawyer to math teacher, happened thanks to Ricky.

The story is this. During my first year at Georgetown, my business classes were not lighting me up, igniting my creativity, or capturing my heart, and I craved those things. Many business students in my Productions and Operations Management class felt the opposite, as if they were in exactly the right place.* But not me. So I looked around for somewhere to channel my energy, and I found Georgetown's Community Outreach Club.

The club's mission was to help out in the urban community, and I was assigned to work at a homework center in downtown DC.

My job was technically to help kids with their homework, which sounds nice, but in reality I spent all my time trying to keep order in the room. Someone else would have been better suited to the job; I imagined a big lovable-but-strict teddy bear of a guy, like the physical therapist character who looks like Sinbad in *Regarding Henry*.

At the homework center, I did, however, make a nice connection with a fifth grader in the group named Ricky. So I was thrilled when Ricky's parents asked me to tutor him outside the program. He was getting old for the group, so they offered to pay me the $35 a week that they had been paying the center if I would come to their house and tutor Ricky after school three days a week.

Ricky and his family lived in a two-room apartment in DC. Not two bedrooms, but two rooms. His mother worked as a house cleaner, and his father was a huge man with giant hands who came home from work every day in a tux. I was convinced that he was low-level muscle for a local crime boss, but I think in reality he drove a limo or maybe bussed dishes in a fancy restaurant.

---

* Actually, to be precise, while some people did feel that way in certain business classes, as if they were in exactly the right place, no one felt that way in Productions and Operations Management class. The professor was horrible, and since attendance was mandatory, students would sign in and then literally crawl out the window when he turned around. One time a friend and I conspired to make a run for the door. When the prof turned, I sprinted. I made it through the door and watched from the hallway as Midge followed. As the prof turned back around to face the class, Midge was caught midstride. She froze, eyes wide, panicked, deer in the headlights, and then she dove, headfirst, Pete Rose–style, through the open door and into the hallway to a standing ovation from the rest of the class. Needless to say, she was a legend after that.

Ricky was a D student and had been labeled by his school a bad kid and future drug user. They had basically written him off.

Ricky had simply been caught between two languages: his family and community spoke Spanish, but he learned English at school. No one at home was able to help him with his homework, and he felt lost in school. Who *doesn't* goof off when they feel lost, frustrated, and trapped? But once he had help with his homework, Ricky worked tirelessly, and his grades soared. I actually became worried that he was caring too much — in fact, he started reminding me quite a bit of myself.

Ricky and I spent many hours together each week. Sometimes on my days off, he'd call with a homework crisis, and I'd stop by for twenty minutes or we'd work together over the phone. Some days I just stopped by for no reason, and we'd hang out.

Ricky and his family were so proud of him, and so appreciative of me. His mom and dad loved me the way only a parent can love a complete stranger who helps their child. They treated me like family. I appreciated the $35 a week, and just as much I loved the homemade paella. A home-cooked meal is priceless to a college student on a meal plan, and even more priceless to a college student on the daily ramen noodles and mac 'n' cheese of a non–meal plan.

Here's how much Ricky's mom loved me: She regularly committed for me the unpardonable sin of cooking paella without pork or beef, and without even understanding why this was necessary. She just went on faith. She'd cook their paella on the traditional paella pan that covers four burners, and on a very sad and lonely electric chafing dish she'd cook my anemic meat-free paella.

My vegetarian desires vexed Ricky's mom to no end, but she simply acquiesced. The pork she easily wrote off to my religion ("*Oh*, es Judeo.") — I believe that I was the first red-blooded, curly-haired, prominent-nosed, honest-to-goodness Jew to enter their home. Ricky's dad once reassured me, "My boss is Whooish, and he's very nice too."

So while Ricky's mom could rationalize my pork ban, she had absolutely no context for understanding my beef abstinence. I think she really worried about me.

The language and culture gap between Ricky's parents and me caused many funny blips. One day I had a cold, and Ricky's mom kept asking me if I was constipated. I assumed she was very nosy or at least very, very holistic, acknowledging the connection between healthy bowel movements and overall well-being. However, in Spanish, "Do you have a cold?" sounds like "¿Estás constipada?" This misunderstanding was not as bad as when in Spain, years later, in my rusty Spanish, I accidentally asked a bartender at a tapas bar for his penis ("¿Puedo tener su polla?"), when all I wanted was the chicken special ("¿Puedo tener su pollo?"). That lowercase *o* can keep you out of jail.

Ricky and I worked together for three years, from fifth through seventh. And at the end of sixth grade, after he had been tutored for two years, Ricky was honored as one of the twenty-five most improved Hispanic students in all of DC. At a formal ceremony, he received a savings bond, a personally signed certificate, and a hug from Washington, DC, mayor Sharon Pratt Dixon.

Ricky was no longer a D student or a "drug risk." On the contrary, he was a straight-A student, a role model, and a class leader.

Ricky went on to great success in middle and high school. Unfortunately, a few years later we lost touch when he moved back to Spain. If you have exceptional Google skills, maybe you can help me find him. I'd love to get back in touch. Trouble is, every third male in Spain is named Ricardo García, and one particularly prominent Flamenco guitarist dominates the first few pages of hits.

My experience with Ricky sold me on teaching. I saw that I had the ability to help children. Plus, working with Ricky felt easy and natural, as if I was built to do it. So when I approached the job search during senior year at Georgetown, I decided to teach.

Being a member of the Georgetown University School of Business Administration senior class, but not planning an illustrious career with Arthur Andersen Consulting (*wink, wink*), put me in a funny situation. Suddenly, for me, all those mixers and dinners and cocktail hours where students networked with corporate recruiters were not sweaty, nerve-racking events, but free eats.

Honestly, I may have been a bit of an ass. I don't know why, perhaps I was delighted to be free of their corporate grip, or maybe I thought I was a bit superior to everyone else in business school, but I'd show up à la Don Johnson in a T-shirt and sport coat. The simple absence of the collared shirt totally changes the outfit and its message at a corporate mixer. Wearing a collared shirt says, "I conform," or at least "I respect you," whereas not wearing it simply says, "Fuck you." I also laughed a bit too loudly and ate food from the buffet like Dan Aykroyd in *Trading Places*. I was even known to wear leather sandals.

If this had been a movie, every recruiter would have been awed by my impertinence and brio and would have begged me to interview. But in reality recruiters probably didn't notice my shenanigans, or if they did, they were probably just annoyed. I was like a drunk person who sees himself as impressive, charming, and witty, but to others just looks like a sweaty Kanye West stealing the mic from Taylor Swift at the 2009 MTV Video Music Awards.

I sent out résumés to every private school in northeastern New Jersey (I did not have a teaching certificate, so I could teach only at private schools). I interviewed with a few math departments and secured a position teaching algebra and geometry in Morristown, New Jersey. The apartment Larry and I found in Jersey City was twenty-five minutes away.

⁂

In Jersey City I found yoga classes being offered at the gym right in my apartment complex. The teacher, Janice, taught a toned-down form of Iyengar yoga, the same style I had practiced during sophomore year of college. This style focuses greatly on correct alignment. Put it this way: in his classic book, *Light on Yoga*, B. K. S. Iyengar includes five hundred pages of instruction and six hundred photographs.

Plus, Mr. Iyengar ranks the difficulty level of every posture. When I first read this book I was flummoxed to discover that the triangle posture, which I found difficult enough, earned a mere three out of a possible sixty, ahead of only a small handful of postures, such as mountain, the one where you stand with your arms overhead, as in, "Touchdown!"

I'm sure you're wondering what Mr. Iyengar ranks as the most difficult yoga posture. It's not the iconic leg-behind-your-head pose (called *eka pada sirsasana*, by the way) made famous by Yogi Kudu on TV's *That's Incredible*.*

To Iyengar, *tiriang mukhottanasana* rings in at a whopping sixty, the most difficult of all yoga postures. *Tiriang mukhottanasana* translates into English as "intense upward-facing pose." Not for the faint of heart, this pose won't be found in a level-one Anusara class. Even its name is no fun, unlike, say, upward dog, boat, or, my favorite, the wind-relieving posture — all child's play at ratings of one, one, and one. Intense upward-facing pose is basically just touching your toes. No biggie, right? But it's touching your toes from the wrong side, bending backward instead of forward. Yep, just bend backward until your hands are at your feet, and there you have a sixty!

---

* On the show, Yogi Kudu would contort his body to fit into a two-foot-square Plexiglas box. Then Cathy Lee Crosby, John Davidson, and Fran Tarkenton would toss the box into a swimming pool or bury him underground for fifteen minutes.

Iyengar yoga, with its specific instructions and meticulous approach to alignment, is very effective in addressing injuries. So I was very lucky to have Janice early that school year, after a skydiving mishap in Southern California.

Let me begin by saying that when you are in a very small airplane halfway to a drop zone, you do not want your jump instructor to say anything like, "*Shit*, I forgot his goggles." And you *definitely* do not want the pilot to answer, "Here, take mine," as he swerves the plane while removing his.

Skydiving enthusiasts are, by definition, very cavalier. They are chill. They do tequila shots after a hard day's work. I have my suspicions they do tequila shots *during* a hard day's work. They're half cowboy, half secret agent. They're probably the toughest and coolest cats on the planet. They make Hawaiian big-wave surfers seem like Urkel.

And I am not like them. I plan. I analyze risk. I don't eat chicken that's more than three days old. I wear a belt from the Gap, for Pete's sake.

But in college, two friends and I had decided to try skydiving. We had all backed out last minute, and so here we were a year later to make good. We met up in Southern California during a long weekend for one purpose: to jump out of an airplane.

Manuel flew to California first and rented a blazing yellow convertible Mazda Miata. He picked me up at the Los Angeles airport and we drove, top down, into the desert. Cordelia, who lived in Fresno, was waiting for us.

To save time and money we opted to jump tandem. That means we'd be strapped to the front of an instructor, like twins conjoined at the genitals. Because we were jumping tandem, we needed almost no instruction. So after signing a seriously long waiver that absolved the skydiving company for an exhaustive number of ways in which we might die, we received basic instruction and were ready to suit up.

My instructor was a slacker, and quite hung over, I believe. He lumbered off to wardrobe to find me a jumpsuit and came back with one that was much too small. But we were running late for the next take-off, so his attitude was "Ve shall make eet fit," as he helped me stuff myself into the suit.

I couldn't stand up straight. I hobbled over to the airplane and grabbed hold of a ceiling bar, and we were off. The plane fit eleven, plus the pilot. And since it was used only for jumps, there was no door.

Here's what I remember. We take off. We get higher and higher. I look around. No door on the plane. The pilot gives me his goggles. Not an auspicious sign.

Cordelia jumps first. Then Manuel. Then it's my turn.

My instructor mounts me. I'm his bitch for the next twenty minutes. We do an odd conjoined dance toward the door. I'm standing at the door, holding on to a railing, and looking down twelve thousand feet. I have never before looked straight down twelve thousand feet. That's more than two miles. If you're standing at the top of the Eiffel Tower and looking over the edge, that's a very safe one thousand feet. We are *twelve times* as high.

We had each paid an extra $80 to have a guy attach a video camera to his head and jump with us. He's standing ready. By law, I have to be the one to jump us from the plane. My instructor can only follow my lead. I steel myself and leap. Obviously the plane is moving, so as soon as I launch, the wind takes over. I forget to tuck, and I kick the videographer in the head.

Fortunately, he's okay.

Now I'm free-falling. I will free-fall for forty-five seconds and travel nine thousand feet in that short time. That means I'm falling at more than 130 miles an hour.

I forget to close my mouth. The airflow makes my cheeks look like Louis Armstrong's. When I say that I forgot to close my mouth, that implies that I had thoughts. I did not.

For those forty-five seconds I receive a mental enema. It washes me clean. Usually I have no less than fifteen simultaneous thoughts, worries, and fears. Here I have only one, in the same way that a mouse being chased by a cat has only one. You could say that it was complete yogic one-pointed concentration.

Then, my instructor starts yelling something at me. I have no idea what he is saying. No idea even, until then, that he and I can communicate. No idea that such a thing is possible. I am primordial soup — precommunicative.

Luckily, though, there is no law that I have to be the one to pull the chute, which he has been shouting at me to do, because he then reaches past me and grabs the dummy cord. We lurch from 130 miles an hour to a leisurely 10 miles an hour. Not good in a jumpsuit that does not fit, and my lower back takes the brunt.

Running on adrenaline, I do not even realize I am hurt until later when I'm seated in Manuel's Miata.

Really, I got off easy. I wasn't hurt too badly. I had to hobble around for a week. I couldn't run for a month. And I got to tell everyone that I had been skydiving — earning me a fair bit of clout with my teen students.

And luckily, Janice was a genius at therapeutic yoga. So two months later, I was completely healed. Well, sort of. I think the injury shook up some things in my lower back and abdomen, because something odd began to happen. In Janice's class I would be enjoying warm-ups and standing postures, but then, when led into belly-down poses (cobra, boat, bow, locust), I would become agitated and emotional and sometimes downright pissed.

I came to expect this and would leave the room for the belly-down postures. I'd take a stroll and then watch from the window to return when I could see Janice had moved on to the shoulder-stand series.

At the time, I did not wonder too much about what was happening; I just knew I was uncomfortable. One moment we're doing mountain posture and I'm focused on my breath and the alignment of my feet and shoulders, and the next we're in cobra, and I'm Fred Flintstone about to blow his top. I was angry at the hard floor, the noisy guy next to me, and even Janice. I blamed them all.

I see now, though, that a great storehouse of stress, agitation, and anger in my gut — I'd say the very angst that had caused the ulcerative colitis — was being tapped and primed for a more thorough release.

In college, I had stretched and relaxed my muscles. I had improved my circulation. I had straightened my posture and improved my diet. I had even experienced periods of mental calm for four or five seconds in a row, and I did not seem to have colitis anymore. And now I was tapping its deeper roots, tapping the twenty years of repressed angst that still lived in my gut.

In new age circles, the kind of circles in which we say things like, "I love your new amber necklace, did you make it?" we call this process of releasing old strains and habits "peeling back the layers of the onion." The idea is that when a layer is removed, a subtler layer underneath is exposed. Stretching and strengthening my muscles and learning to deal with stress had eliminated the outer layer of colitis. Removing that layer had exposed the subtler roots underneath — my habit of repressing angst and storing it in my belly — the root cause of the disease.

When the roots are exposed, yoga helps to eliminate them. It's like pressing on a knotted muscle in your back. Most of the day you might just say, "My back feels stiff." But when you give the muscles a little massage and feel around, you find a knot. When you identify this knot as the source or epicenter of the stiffness, you open up a possibility for its release.

If you press right on the knot and breathe and wait and breathe and watch, you'll find that eventually you sigh or moan or laugh or cry, and the knot releases a little bit or even completely. That's what yoga was doing for the tension in my gut. It had identified the source knot in my belly, and it was pressing right on it (literally, in cobra, boat, bow, and locust postures). Eventually I'd be sighing, moaning, laughing, and mostly crying as it released. But not for another year or so.

In the meantime, my discomfort in Janice's class during belly-down postures eventually passed. I chalked it up to getting stronger and therefore less frustrated as I attempted the postures. And I think that was true, but I also think that my body had done its work accessing and unveiling the tension for the time being and was waiting for the right time to unleash it.

The body really does possess a kind of intelligence, such as the ability to wait for the right time to unleash. Think about how you can wait until you are alone in the bathroom to bawl after a big confrontation at work. Or imagine you're on your way home from work and sense the stirrings of a very large bowel movement. Haven't you ever noticed that your urge grows as you get closer to home? Unless you've got a stomach bug, it never gets unbearable until you're within range of the bathroom.* Now, that's pretty intelligent, if you ask me. So my body knew that this was not the time to unload my angst. Not yet.

---

* I once saw a car with a bumper sticker that read "I'm only speeding 'cause I really have to poop."

Chapter 5

O'Malley's Mushroom Caps

I spent a year teaching in a boy's prep school and that
was a crowd that was trying to make up their minds....
I've seen them since, and those who followed their zeal,
their bliss, they have led decent, wonderful lives;
those who did what [others] said they should do
because it's safe found out it's not safe. It's disaster.

— JOSEPH CAMPBELL, *The Hero's Journey*

I liked teaching, and I loved the kids, but I was bored by the math. It was actually driving me mad. One day I was at the chalkboard teaching side-angle-side proofs for congruent triangles in my third geometry class of the day, and I lost it. I started laughing and couldn't stop. I had to leave the room and ask a student to take over.

While I was bored to tears by my seven hours of math every day, my colleagues could get worked into a tizzy, giggling like schoolkids, about a new fractals poster for the math building hallway.

I believe that we each have a calling and that it is our job to find it. The calling can be to teach math, practice medicine, build schools in India, raise a family, trade stocks, or whatever. Me? I wanted to eat, sleep, and breathe yoga. So at the end of that school year, I left the math job.

At the same time, my brother, Larry, got married and moved in with his wife, Pam, so with our other roommate, Minsheng, I moved across the train tracks to Hoboken, New Jersey. The town of Hoboken is one square mile and rumored to be more densely packed than Calcutta, India. And in 1995 downtown Hoboken was densely packed with recent business school grads who worked in Manhattan but lived in Hoboken for one-fourth the rent.

Downtown Hoboken is essentially the five blocks of town nearest the PATH trains, which go under the Hudson River to bring you two thousand feet to Manhattan. Minsheng commuted daily to the World Financial Center (across the street from where the Twin Towers of the World Trade Center used to stand) and often commented that he could nearly hit a golf ball across the river to his office, yet his one-and-a-half-laps-around-the-track commute could take more than thirty minutes.

To make money I began tutoring math and also waiting tables at a chain restaurant. The tutoring paid pretty well, so the waiting was really just for some extra cash and to hang out with people, because at 7:30 every weekday morning, all the other residents of my newly renovated apartment building got dressed in starched suits, waited in line at Starbucks, and boarded trains to Manhattan, leaving me alone in a ghost town.

All the artists and yogis of Hoboken lived eleven blocks north near the YMCA or seven blocks west in five-story walk-up apartments rented from long-time natives of the Polish district. (The Polish district was legit and still hosted a yearly parade of parishioners hoisting bleeding-saint statues on their shoulders.)

So I needed something social, something to connect me with the other daytime denizens of Hoboken — the artists, the yogis, the out-of-work actors. The restaurant job was perfect for that, though at first I stank at the job. I was attentive and could make diners feel very at home, but waiting on five tables at once left me mixing up orders, bringing soup after main course, serving cold food, and mumbling to myself as I paced the restaurant in a cold sweat.

I might not have been so bad, but on the first day the manager accidentally scheduled me for the busiest section of tables, thinking that I was the other, far more experienced Brian who worked at the restaurant. So on my first day, I was juggling six tables and everything went wrong. Guests were going to the kitchen counter to pick up their own food, and one guy returned his coffee cup four times because I kept bringing cups that were dirty.

I enjoyed the social aspect of the job, but I never really became one of the gang. It takes time, and I was only there for a few months. Not only that, but I was different from these folks. They waited tables, auditioned for roles, and partied at night. I worked the lunch shift, then drove thirty minutes to suburban New Jersey to tutor all afternoon, and went home to upscale, downtown Hoboken to hang out with my Georgetown friends. I had no SAG card, no tattoos, and no criminal record. I was a bit square compared to everyone else at the restaurant.

Being a waiter did afford me some power to make people happy, though, and I enjoyed that. One day at one of my tables I had a bunch of twenty-somethings who were clearly very high. They were hungry the way only marathon runners and pot smokers can be, and when they all emptied out their pockets they came up with only $7.25, so they ordered the nachos appetizer. I brought the nachos and watched them devour it. At this restaurant when it was someone's birthday we could comp them a beautiful brownie sundae, so I clicked the button on the register for a birthday sundae. When I presented it to them, it was Christmas in O'Malley's. I bet they still tell stories of that unexpected, fully loaded sundae in 1994.

Even though this job basically fit my need to interact with human beings during the daytime hours, I was growing uneasy with it. In my personal life, I was doing a lot of yoga and beginning to study natural health. Meanwhile, at O'Malley's, I was dishing out platter after platter of deep-fried calamari, oily French fries, and fried stuffed mushrooms. Plus, O'Malley's was a chain, so all the food was prepared at the mother ship in Texas and delivered weekly, and who knows what additives and fillers were in those five-gallon tubs o' processed gloop.

I grew increasingly uncomfortable and guilty, and eventually I felt that I could no longer in good conscience shop for myself at the Hoboken natural foods market and dish out O'Malley's food to others. I know that people ate there of their own accord, and that there are worse things in the world than deep-fried mushroom caps, but I could no longer eat one kind of way and serve food that represented another. Plus, I wanted to grow a beard. (At O'Malley's, workers were not allowed to have facial hair.)

One day a friend came to visit from Virginia, and I wanted to spend time with her. I canceled my shift that day and was told that I'd need a doctor's note to return to work. I had no note, so it was essentially like quitting. To celebrate, I grew a big beard that would have made Dr. Andrew Weil, Oskar from Georgetown, and even Zach Galifianakis proud.

I have since found that feeling good about my work is absolutely crucial to my happiness. When I work a job that is out of line with my values, I become depressed, and when I am in dharma, following my heart, doing what I believe in and what feels right, I am filled with energy.

The Buddha called this "right livelihood." He taught that one who seeks liberation cannot hope to find freedom on the backs of others. Right livelihood is critical to the spiritual path; often when people are out of line with their values they have to numb out or shut down, not only because they are bored and uninterested but also because the pain of being outside their morals or their heart's call is too much to bear. Interestingly, yoga brings these issues to the surface. Many times I have seen students of yoga realize that their job is hurting them. Sometimes making a change is too much to face. In these cases, people usually stop practicing yoga, and the revelation fades.

One time I was in a new relationship and had moved far away

from New Jersey to be with my girlfriend. I had been practicing yoga consistently for years, but without even noticing, I gave it up. A month later, browsing in a bookstore, I stumbled onto a quote from yoga teacher Dr. Jeff Migdow: "When people do yoga consistently they're much more open to change. That's the key: If I'm not open to making changes, then I won't let myself be aware."

The quote was a slap in the face. As if waking from a daze, I realized that I had not done postures in a month. And I saw that I had avoided yoga because it sharpened my awareness and showed me that I was unhappy. But because I had been unwilling to make a change — to move and leave the relationship — I had stopped doing the thing that increased my awareness. In this way, yoga is a catalyst that demands truth.

This truth includes, but is also subtler than, simply doing what is right or wrong, ethical or moral. It means listening to your heart's call.

I love to share this with my tutoring students. I remember a student, Aidan, was considering college majors and said, "I'd love to be an architect, but the world needs environmental activists, so that's what I'll do."

Aidan is correct. We do need environmental activists. But I believe that even more, we need people who are passionate about what they do, living from their heart. I don't think one can actually serve the world best by assessing what the world needs. I think, instead, we serve the world best by responding to our heart's call. Not our ego's call, mind you, but our heart's.

As an environmental activist, Aidan might make a difference. That's true. But as an architect, Aidan will be following his bliss. He'll be fulfilled and happy. He'll be lit up and creative. He'll be a beacon of light and energy. And, I trust, his environmental concerns will still find a very effective, perhaps more effective, medium — maybe he'll design green buildings or discover environmentally sustainable building materials.

Joseph Campbell told his students, "If you do follow your bliss, you put yourself on a kind of track that has been there all the while, waiting for you, and the life that you ought to be living is the one you are living...Wherever you are — if you are following your bliss, you are enjoying that refreshment, that life within you, all the time."

And so, in our spiritual Easter egg hunt for the Keys to Happiness, we come to key number two:

Follow your heart.

Notice what gives you a feeling of rightness, ignites your creativity and passion, and makes you feel most alive, and pursue that.

Before every major decision, ask yourself, "Which choice feels right, is in line with my values, ignites my creativity and passion, and is an expression of my true self?"

And by the way, following your bliss does not automatically mean giving up your nine-to-five job at the insurance company to dust off your old Fender Stratocaster and get the college funk band back together. Sometimes the boring job at the insurance company is just right. Your bliss might be the paycheck that feeds your family and allows you to spend happy evenings and weekends together. Or not. Following your bliss only means tuning in to and following not your ego, not your mind, but your heart. Put another way, it means setting aside what you want and doing what God* wants for you. And God, I believe, communicates through our hearts and through a feeling of passion, vitality, and rightness.

---

* When I say God, I'm referring to my belief in an intelligent, benevolent energy that permeates, sustains, and guides reality. If, for you, this definition rings a bit too close to the *Shit New Age Guys Say* YouTube videos, you can swap in the words *love, goddess, prana, Jesus, Tim Tebow,* or *Ralph Nader.* Whatever floats your boat.

Chapter 6

Kripalu Yoga

Take the attitude that what you are thinking and feeling
is valuable stuff.

— ANNE LAMOTT, *Bird by Bird*

*D*ifferent types of people, with different constitutions and dis-positions, can find what they need in one of the various yoga styles. Power yoga makes you feel more, well, powerful and gives you a heck of a workout. Iyengar yoga makes you feel embodied and correct. And Kripalu yoga makes you feel, well, you'll see.

I don't think there's a formula for which style will speak to a practitioner any more than there is a formula for who will fall in love. Match.com can put you in touch with people who share your interests, but you have to date to see if there's chemistry. We can say, "Aha, you like a vigorous workout, try Power yoga," but ultimately you have to date a few styles to see which one ignites your passion. And that passion, just like the chemistry of love, is quite magical and special and transformational.

In Hoboken I stumbled onto that kind of chemistry with a style of yoga being offered around the corner from my apartment in the attic of a natural foods market. Shopping at the store on a Saturday, I spotted a flyer for "Yoga with Yolanthe."

The Hoboken Harvest was an old-school health food store —

the only kind of health food store in 1994 — the kind that existed before Whole Foods Market introduced Newman-O's to mainstream Americans. Before Whole Foods propagated the concept of the whole foods supermarket, health food stores were small, purely organic, and dusty. They carried only organic produce, though the produce was kept in substandard conditions, making it either half-frozen or wilty. The stores smelled of the unmistakable combination of patchouli and vitamins, and had small cafés operated by idealist vegans.

The café of the Hoboken Harvest was run by a fellow by the name of Guy. I had a real-life Abbot and Costello conversation when I asked someone at the store, "What's the name of the guy who runs the café?"

"Guy."

"Yes, the guy who runs the café."

"Guy."

This Guy was a character, a Vietnam War veteran turned vegan who, like every health food store café operator in 1994, was not shy about sharing his political opinions, espousing his conspiracy theory, or selling you a share in his blue-green algae distribution network. I miss those places. My aunt has been a vitamin-taking, patchouli-burning, macrobiotic-eating meditator since the 1970s, and her apartment somehow carries a hint of that original health food store smell and vibe. It makes my muscles melt and my heart open every time I smell it.

The yoga classes were held in the attic of the Harvest. The showroom of the Harvest was dusty, so you might expect the attic to be a nightmare, but local yoga teacher and longtime Hoboken resident (she lived uptown with the artists and yogis near the YMCA) Yolanthe Smit had co-opted this space and made it lovely. She cleaned it assiduously. She draped beautiful Indian scarves and tapestries, she burned incense (only before class so it would scent the room but not interfere with our yogic breathing exercises), she changed the lighting, and she created an altar. She even played CDs of bamboo flutes and birds chirping as we practiced. It was a sanctuary.

I attended Yolanthe's classes three times a week. Her classes were called Kripalu (meaning "compassion") yoga, named for Swami Kripalu, the guru of Amrit Desai, who founded the Kripalu Center for Yoga and Health in Massachusetts.

Amrit was called at that time Gurudev, meaning "beloved guru," and he was ever present in the class — on a poster demonstrating the yoga postures and on the altar at the front of the room.

I loved everything about the class. I loved the smell of the sati incense. I loved the music and the altar and the pictures of Gurudev. I loved that the class began and ended with chanting "om," and that we shared with the group about our day. I loved that we were led to ignite and follow our own body's guidance and wisdom as we practiced. I loved that we were invited to "sound" and emote. To sound basically means to moan, either from the blissful pain of the stretch or from the release of tension or emotion that a posture might trigger.

I even loved my walk to class — I felt like an insider, a member of a secret society as I marched straight through the store, past the tofu pies and organic black bean corn chips, and headed for the back stairs. I'd nod to Guy, keeper of the stairs, as he polished his counter or mindfully flipped a Sunshine burger. I felt like part of something, or even part of a revolution, attending secret insurgent meetings in the attic of the Harvest. In a way I was an insurgent, at least in the minds of my parents and my Georgetown business school friends.

Yolanthe's class captured my spirit in a way no other class had. I loved Oskar's Sivananda yoga class at Georgetown. I loved Janice's Iyengar yoga class at the gym in Jersey City. But Kripalu yoga gave me permission to be me. It invited the *whole* me to show up, and really, I'd say that was the first time that the whole me had been invited anywhere.

A typical class in the attic of the Harvest started with all of us sitting cross-legged in a circle and the following introduction, called a "centering," by Yolanthe:

"Close your eyes and tune in to your body. (*pause*) Notice your buttocks on the ground. (*pause*) Notice your clothes resting on your body. (*pause*) Feel your belly rise and fall with each breath. (*longer pause*) Notice when your mind wanders away to think about lunch, work, or your to-do list, and bring it back to this room — to feeling your body, your belly rising and falling with each breath. (*long pause*) For today, for the next hour and fifteen minutes, give yourself permission to be fully here in this class with nothing else to do and nowhere else to be — nothing else to accomplish but paying attention to your body and hearing its messages, for the next hour and fifteen minutes. (*long pause*) *Ahohhhmmmm. Ahohhhmmmm. Ahohhhmmmm.*"

Sometimes I'd hear the whole intro. Mostly my mind wandered off, uncontrollably reviewing my morning or planning my afternoon, and I'd hear Yolanthe's voice faintly in the background. But I loved the idea and the intention.

Occasionally, I actually succeeded in giving myself permission to be only there. Sometimes I could set aside planning and problem solving until after class. No one had ever asked me to do this before. And no one had ever asked me to listen to what my body was telling me.

At first I tackled this project with the same diligence and anxiety I had used throughout school. I was obsessed. "I'm listening to my body...I'm listening to my body...Oh, I think I feel the stirrings of a pee! Better go." I'd get up, tiptoe around everyone in their frog postures, and head to the bathroom to pee. Three drops.

Later, I'd realize, "Oh, wait a minute, I think I might be cold! Better put on my sweater."

I wanted an A in this assignment. Plus, I was asking my body, for the first time, what it wanted, and like a six-year-old who's allowed to chew gum for the first time, my body wanted a mouthful.

And my body and I, as new acquaintances, needed some time to get to know each other. I had not had this type of consciousness before. In fact, I'd say that this lack of body consciousness had contributed to my colitis. If I was stiff, I didn't think to stretch. If I was stressed, I didn't think to take a few deep breaths. I just ignored all that. And if my head hurt from studying or if my stomach hurt during a debate tournament, I didn't think to take a break; I just popped some Tylenol or downed some Pepto and kept going.

I became quite fond of Yogi Amrit Desai as he sat blissfully framed on the altar and in his poster demonstrating *janu-shirshasana* (head-to-knee forward bend). He had created Kripalu yoga, and to me he represented this new sanctuary I had found.

Interestingly, I believe that fate protected me from meeting famous yogis back in those days. I was a *sadhak*, a seeker, and I was young, idealistic, and impressionable. Fate kept me from meeting any big-name charismatic spiritual teachers. I'd attend a retreat or visit a center and miss the guru or a visiting swami by a day. I think this worked to my advantage. I wonder if I would have given away everything and joined up full tilt with the first guru I met.

Yolanthe, however was a perfect and safe emissary of Amrit's teachings. She did not seek to be revered. She just lived as she saw fit, and that included teaching yoga. Yolanthe was very authentic. She was also opinionated, and she was very strong, a bulldog in many ways. In fact, whereas many members of the extended Kripalu community from around the world would go to Kripalu to assist programs as a way to visit the ashram for free, Yolanthe had been banned from assisting at Kripalu. Don't get me wrong — she had a huge heart and was a terrific friend. It was the program directors who had banned her. I doubt a guest in a program ever had a problem with her, but if she disagreed with how a director led a program, while other assistants would keep quiet, Yolanthe would speak up. And that was actually against the rules. Directors are under a lot of pressure, and assistants are not supposed to criticize. Honestly, I think that was a lame rule, one endemic of certain problems with authenticity at Kripalu in those days, but anyway, that is why Yolanthe was banned from assisting. She was like *Seinfeld*'s Kramer, banned from the fruit stand for bringing back a subpar peach.

She and I became buddies — not teacher and disciple, just friends. We'd discuss enlightenment over lunch, attend esoteric talks, and ride the ferry across the Hudson River to Rollerblade in New York City's World Financial Center. I had felt misplaced in the 1980s and 1990s, as if I had been cheated and placed in the wrong decade. But Yolanthe brought me back. She spoke freely of yoga, spirit, God, business, art, food, orgasms, and masturbation, as though these were all perfectly normal parts of the human experience.

Then, one day in October 1994, after I had been taking her classes at the Harvest religiously for five months, Yolanthe came in and laid out the news. "Amrit Desai," she said, "has been asked to leave Kripalu. He is accused of abusing his power and having affairs with several disciples."

I was pretty crushed. Though I had never met him, Amrit had become my de facto guru. I had even been planning to live at the ashram for a monthlong Kripalu yoga teacher training.

How could I follow a guru who had hurt so many people? If Amrit Desai had mastered yoga's postures and practices yet still committed these transgressions, what could yoga offer me? And especially Amrit Desai's yoga? Would his flawed fingerprint taint the very tenets of Kripalu yoga?

I decided to stop practicing yoga entirely.

BOOK TWO

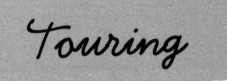
Touring

Chapter 7

Tea with Oskar

Not all those who wander are lost.

— GANDALF, in *The Fellowship of the Ring*

After hearing about Amrit, I still tutored, I still hung out with Yolanthe; I just didn't do yoga anymore.

Until I did. One day, only a few days after my yoga ban, I realized that I was in the middle of a yoga practice. I was not asleep or drugged; I was just doing yoga, in much the same manner that you'd eventually breathe if you had been holding your breath. You'd get distracted by something and find that there you were, of course, breathing. That's what happened to me. I got distracted, so to speak, and suddenly found that there I was, practicing yoga.

Around the same time that Yolanthe told me the devastating Amrit news, one of my oldest and closest friends was talking about traveling. Like me, Zach was at a crossroads and needed some time to think. His questions were different from mine — while my disillusionment sprang from a wayward guru, Zach's centered on several early professional disappointments, a broken heart, and a very bad sunburn.*

But for both of us, traveling seemed a way to find some answers.

Zach and I spent a few months doing research. First we decided to travel the United States rather than Europe. Second, we decided to buy a van rather than patch together trains and buses across the country.

I figured that on the trip I would experiment with yoga styles and find the one for me. I even found a few directories of yoga schools and teachers in the United States. It would be like speed dating after a rough breakup.

Zach located a van for us to buy. We had almost settled on a retired Wonder Bread delivery truck, but instead we purchased a 1990 Toyota Previa minivan. We removed the backseats and replaced them with a futon. We designed the futon frame to lift at both ends so we could store our stuff underneath.

On March 8, my parents threw a good-bye party for us. It was a heck of a scene. You will fail to visualize this event properly unless you have witnessed fifteen elderly New Jersey Jews passing around plates of pastrami and dill pickles and talking all at once. My paternal grandpa struggled to understand the *mishegas* of his grandson. He had no chance at understanding why two *menschly* fellows like Zach and I were "not in med school, *already*!" My mom cried as we pulled away in the van.

Our first stop was a pilgrimage for me. I wanted answers, and I thought perhaps Oskar, the guy in sandals, beard, and all whites

---

* The sunburn, often blamed for the broken heart, involved a very botched trip to the beach after his senior-year spring formal. You'll soon learn about Ayurveda, and let's just say that Zach is very *pitta*, so seven hours in the North Carolina sun turns Zach a mighty painful crimson color and leaves him in no condition to consummate a relationship.

from Georgetown, could provide them. He had seemed so pure and so yogic. Plus, he had been my very first yoga teacher.

Luckily Oskar was listed in the *Yoga Journal* directory. He taught and lived, it seemed, in Bethesda, Maryland, about twenty minutes from Georgetown. I felt about him the way a kindergartener feels about his teacher; seeing Oskar anywhere else but at yoga class, say, in a CVS wearing jeans and a polo shirt, would have me staring wide-eyed and openmouthed.

I called ahead to ask if I could visit, and then dropped Zach off at a bookstore. I found Oskar's place, and at first the whole experience was perfect, textbook. He had an old VW bus parked in the driveway. I rang the bell, which was short and sweet, a cross between a Zen chime and a gong.

Oskar opened the door and looked just as I remembered him: relaxed smile, comfortable white clothing, big beard, sandals, as if no time had passed. Really very little had passed, but to me the time between my graduation from college and now, which had been only two years, was significant. To him, in midlife, it probably didn't seem like very long.

Oskar pointed me to the family room, while he went to the kitchen for mugs of ginger tea. We chatted, first catching up and then getting down to business. I told him about Kripalu yoga, the news about Amrit (he knew of this already), my disillusionment, and my attempts to stop practicing yoga.

Oskar listened attentively. After I was finished, he started dishing out some very fine wisdom. He spoke in metaphor and parable. He told me that when the bee stings the deer (an interesting metaphor for Amrit's sexual indiscretions), the bee is acting out its nature. And best of all, he told me that my attempts at quitting yoga, which ended with me unconsciously taking the practice right back up, demonstrated that I had been practicing for many lifetimes and that it was my dharma, my work in this lifetime, to pursue yoga and liberation. I was an old, wise soul, he said.

I sat and listened. I was enthralled. Who doesn't want to hear that they are an old, wise soul? And then suddenly I noticed that Oskar's eyes were half closed as he spoke. I remembered that three years earlier, someone at Georgetown, who was doing a research paper on enlightenment, had told me that an enlightened person is so relaxed that their eyes are always half closed.

I was elated, ebullient, ecstatic, euphoric — exultant, even. I had done it. I had met a living master. On the very first stop of the trip, I had found my new style of yoga, *and* my guru. And better than in a fairy tale, he had been my very first teacher. It was kismet, and he was dishing out the good news, right there in the flesh.

It was a dream come true.

As our visit was coming to a close, I told him, "I'll be in town for a few days, and would love to attend your class at Georgetown while I'm here." I could just see it, lead disciple returns to the master, like Luke returning to Yoda, Darth returning to Obi Wan, Harry returning to Dumbledore, Ari Gold returning to Terrance McQuewick. I was ready to give it all away: "Zach, thanks for a great trip. I've found what I needed. Enjoy the van."

But instead of inviting me to join (or hopefully lead) his class, instead of asking me to be a disciple, instead of ordaining me with a Sanskrit name and anointing me as his successor right then and there, Oskar said, in his unmistakable baritone that made his guided relaxations so velvety, "Brian, I'd love for you to come to class, but I just had cataract surgery, and the doctor won't let me teach for another two weeks. Plus, with these darn drops in my eyes, I can barely see."

And actually, I was not disappointed. I was happily disillusioned — another reminder that, at that time, for me, the goal was not to find a guru, but to find me. As Amrit was famous for saying, "Your *own* body is the best expert on yoga you will ever find."

Chapter 8

Fearless, Honest, Relaxed

Life moves pretty fast. If you don't stop and look around
once in a while, you could miss it.

— FERRIS BUELLER, *Ferris Bueller's Day Off*

Our next stop was Chapel Hill, North Carolina. Zach wanted us
to check in with his University of North Carolina sociology
professor, Richard Anderson. I had had my pilgrimage, and I think
this was Zach's. Zach called ahead to let Richard know we were on
our way.

We showed up just after 6:00 PM. A girl there was in tears, hugging Richard and thanking him for his help. Richard was a UNC
legend, part prof, part social worker, part mentor. Even after my
still-fresh Oskar-is-enlightened miscalculation, my mind was sizing
up Richard as potential guru material.

We set up in the den. A fire burned. There was incense in the
air. His wife brought in his dinner — a large plate of lima beans and
brown rice, a beautiful and simple dinner for a man of wisdom. The
beans and rice were not mixed together, but each occupied half the
plate, and if I squinted I could faintly make out a yin-yang symbol.

Richard asked us about our trip and listened as he ate. When he
finished his simple fare, he picked up a guitar and strummed as we
chatted. Richard could easily have subbed for any charismatic cult

leader. He was so captivating that I was actually a bit wary. Give me a weird-looking bearded hippie anytime, but right or wrong, it's the handsome, sparkly-eyed, charismatic types that send up red flags for me. Or maybe I was just a bit jaded after the Amrit business and too many David Koresh made-for-TV movies.

But Richard was wonderful. He spoke of his life. He told us about when he had lived alone on the seaside in Brazil. He'd go to town once a month for a sack of beans and a sack of brown rice. He'd shit in the sea and wash his ass in the waves, no toilet paper.

"People wipe way too far in, you know, it's not healthy," he shared. I felt enlightened and violated all at once. You know I'm a sucker for anyone who's liberated around poop.

I was equally inspired by Richard's lifestyle. I had always wondered how I would ever be ready to settle down, get married, have kids, and earn a living. Richard had done all that, but he had taken his time to get there. He had floated, experimented, and traveled, figuring out how to live, before returning to school for a PhD in sociology. Now at forty, he had been married for two years and had a one-year-old baby.

Perhaps there was hope for me to one day rejoin society and lead the life — getting married, owning a house, and having children — that my parents dreamed for me. Truth be told, I dreamed of it too, but until then, I just didn't see how I'd be ready by the time most people did it. Now I had the potential for a revised timeline. I knew I had to do some exploring, and I knew that I needed time to work some things out and get comfortable in my own skin before I could settle down.

Richard also spoke of his many trips cross-country, and he gave us some advice. If you're twenty-two years old and planning a trip cross-country, lots of people give you advice. But Richard's advice was like spiritual counsel, not just tips on how to get laid or stay alive if we met hillbillies named Festus in Georgia or desperados named Little Bill while crossing the Rockies. His advice was much better than, for example, the advice we received from Zach's uncle who told us to "pack some heat in case you get into a pickle out West."

Richard told us that traveling is an opportunity to live as you want to, an opportunity to experiment with new ways of being and thinking. It's a clean start. You leave behind those who know you, you leave behind your job, you leave behind those who expect your habitual patterns. It's an opportunity to begin anew, to be reborn.

Richard was spot-on for us. Zach and I both were seeking, and we saw this trip as a pilgrimage into our deeper selves, a pilgrimage in search of answers to the questions of who we were and how we should be in the world.

Richard told us that when he and his brother traveled, they had three rules:

1. Be brave. Why stick to the same old ways of being? If that's all you wanted, you'd have stayed home. Try new things.
2. Be honest. People know when you're being honest, and they'll open up to you. You'll find yourself in much more interesting experiences.
3. Stay relaxed. Have fun.

Richard's advice made terrific sense to me. This experience was an opportunity to play with new ways of being, to reinvent myself, to be the man I wanted to be. And it was an opportunity to turn up my level of consciousness a few notches. Without the routine of a daily grind, without a job, without the stress of needing to make rent, things like doing laundry, finding a place to shower, eating a meal, having a walk in the woods, or even meeting a new friend become the focus of the day. I could be more awake to the moments of life as my life simplified.

Richard's advice inspired me, and his rules became my mantra on the trip. Whenever I was afraid, whenever I wanted to fall back on old, established patterns, whenever I found myself in unfamiliar territory on that trip, I'd say to myself, "Fearless, honest, relaxed."

What a way to live. *Fearless* and strong. *Honest* and true. *Relaxed* and at ease. These three intentions synergize beautifully;

they have perfect checks and balances. If *fearless* tells me to jump from a ledge, *honest* can say, "Hey, now, that'll hurt." And if *honest* gets too uptight about some nitty-gritty, let's say, for example, about a girlfriend's new but brutally botched haircut, *relaxed* can say, "She doesn't need *that* much truth, not right now."*

"Fearless, honest, relaxed" is more balanced than that. It helps me break through barriers, try new things, and be the man I want to be, but without being a jerk. I seek to follow my true calling, my inner wisdom, my intuition, and the flow of energy, but not to be a heedless ass or an aggressive jerk. When I have a crush on a girl, "fearless, honest, relaxed," I ask her out. That's how I met my wife. When a friend has been living in his parents' basement for two years too long, "fearless, honest, relaxed," I call him on it. When a parent of a student is pushing too hard, I bring it up. Not just fearless, not just honest, but fearless, honest, *and* relaxed.

On our trip cross-country, luckily, Zach and I never met threatening hillbillies or dark desperados, and we never found ourselves in an unfortunate wooded glen amid a three-county KKK meeting, so I never regretted omitting from my backpack the "heat" that Zach's uncle had recommended. But "fearless, honest, relaxed" got me into some very interesting and transformational situations indeed, like, for example, during our next stop in High Point, North Carolina, at Ruby's massage parlor.

---

* In an earlier incarnation of personal mantras and strict adherence to yogic laws, I decided for a time to be 100 percent radically honest all the time, and during that time I did actually encounter the dreaded, clichéd question, "Does my butt look big?" from a girlfriend. She was in law school and was eating a lot of junk during study sessions, and the honest answer was undeniably "yes." Needless to say, "yes" did not go over very well at all, and I now know "yes" is never *actually* the correct answer.

Chapter 9

Ruby's

[Raja Yoga] is a way to God
through psychophysical experiments.

— HUSTON SMITH, *The Illustrated World's Religions*

Our next stop was High Point, North Carolina. Zach had a buddy there we could stay with for a few days. Zach had been an a cappella singer while in college, with the University of North Carolina Clef Hangers, and for our road trip, the group basically translated into a series of free Clef Hangers youth hostels scattered about the country.

When I wasn't sampling yoga styles, I practiced on my own, and I planned to do so outdoors whenever possible. But I had also hatched a plan for how to practice indoors when it rained or was too cold. Before we set out, Zach and I had signed up for a membership at a gym in New Jersey. The gym belonged to a nationwide network that gave traveling members reciprocal privileges. I imagine that the Council of Gyms and Spas had devised this plan with traveling businesspeople in mind, rather than, say, the unwashed cross-country transient set, but either way, it worked beautifully for us too. The gyms gave me a place to do yoga on rainy days, and they gave us a place to catch a shower (and usually even a Jacuzzi) in most major towns across the country.

Sometimes, especially out West, where towns are farther apart, the location of the nearest gym decided where we were headed. The need to shower can sneak up on you. One moment all is well, and then in the next, the feeling of accumulated sweat and grime becomes too much to bear, and you're overcome by an itchy, agitated angst and *must have a shower, now!*

These days, in my busy daily life of working, exercising, doing chores, and raising kids (which involves being vomited on and regularly having bubbles spilled all over me, not to mention the obvious involvement with at least three different people's tushie wipings each day), I find it difficult to imagine not enjoying my daily hot shower. Maybe I've gone soft, but on the trip I could go a solid five days before the urge arrived. When it did, though, as I mentioned, it was fierce. So we'd check the reciprocal gym membership directory and plot our course to the nearest participating gym. The directory also listed the gym's amenities, so given the choice between two equally close gyms, we'd always select the one with the Jacuzzi and the free fruit.

Along with the shower, Jacuzzi, and fruit, I'd also find a space to do yoga. In even the most old-school, boxing-ring-in-the-corner type of gym, I could practice postures on the mat in the free-weights warm-up area. This area can be pretty intimidating, though, full of testosterone, hair gel, and the guys from *Jersey Shore*. Imagine a tall, thin vegetarian, with a mighty thick beard, bending himself into unnatural positions among Ronnie and Pauly D, as well as Hans, Franz, and Arnie: "Who is dis girlie man in revolved triangle posture?"

The Hans and Franz free-weight gyms were actually better than the upscale gyms with attendants in the bathroom handing out aftershave, where I feared getting run out of town.

The best gyms for my yoga comfort had a semiprivate aerobics room. This was 1995, so unless we were in Asheville, North

Carolina, or Boulder, Colorado, I did not count on the gym having a dedicated yoga space. I suspect that now most large gyms have a full lineup of yoga classes and perhaps even a specialized yoga room, but back then at gyms in Des Moines, Texarkana, Butztown, Dinosaur Footprints, Pig Eye, or Tupelo, I was just happy to hunker down in a semiprivate aerobics room.

On this particular rainy day in High Point, Zach was out with his college buddy, Howard, and I was ready to do some yoga. Howard's apartment was lovely, but his overly amicable cats and doorless open-floor-plan apartment made yoga in his flat impossible. I could have practiced right there on the den floor — and I'm sure to receive angry, instructive letters regarding where to stick it from avid cat-fan yogis on this one (and there are many, many avid cat-fan yogis) — but I could not do yoga there. I would have been on constant alert, expecting a cat ass at any moment to plant itself gingerly on my face and yank me from my yoga reverie. I can palpably feel it right now. First the slightest tickle and itch of cat fur feathering my nostrils, and then boom, cat ass, smack-dab right on my open mouth.

This extremely rational fear would have prevented me from sinking deeply into any kind of yoga posture or meditation. My sister-in-law, a cat lover, knew of my feelings on this matter and threatened to tuck catnip into my beard when I slept at their place. I'd have woken from some licentious dream to find Shorty cat eagerly humping my beard.

All this cat business reminds me of a time when I was visiting my aunt in Florida. She is a Yorkie person and always has at least two tiny Yorkshire terriers prancing about her apartment. As a child I was terrified of the dogs. I think to a small child, tiny dogs are probably more frightening than huge ones. Huge dogs are simply out of children's league, like those beings in *Star Trek* that move so fast humans can't even see them. We could occupy the same room and never know they were there. But little dogs are realistic rivals for a child, and they have claws and make a terrible noise.

As I got older, I made peace with the dogs. Perhaps I grew braver or more accustomed to them, or perhaps as I grew larger, they grew cuter. Plus, unlike Howard's cats, these small dogs like their privacy and keep a distance from strangers. But on one visit, while my aunt and uncle were out, I was lying on the floor in relaxation pose at the end of a yoga practice, and Rocky came over and started licking my bare foot. You know that some dog tongues are like sandpaper, so this small dog licking my foot felt like having a tiny expert massage therapist wearing an expensive exfoliating glove and oh so gently stroking my foot. He got into all the nooks — the arch, between the toes. It was luscious. I lay there and let him have at it.

I just assumed that Rocky was getting something from our union as well. Why else would he be doing it? Maybe he was a bit dehydrated and needed the salt from my foot, or maybe he needed some tongue workout — who knows — but I assumed I could trust nature (I forgot about the whole dogs-will-eat-until-they-get-sick phenomenon).

After some time, perhaps ten minutes, I was feeling a bit imbalanced. I needed a little love for the right foot. Careful not to break his concentration (and he was ridiculously and zealously concentrated — which should have been my tip-off that all was not well here), I slid my right foot next to my left foot and transitioned Rocky from licking my left to licking my right.

Ten minutes later I was balanced and had the most relaxed (and cleanest) feet in the state. I showered up, got dressed, went to the beach for the day, and thought nothing more of it...until dinner, when my aunt in casual conversation said with a confused look on her face, "I still don't know why Rocky was throwing up all afternoon. I don't think it's something he ate."

For the rest of the dinner I made sure to have my mouth full at all times so that I was neither available for questioning nor able to turn myself in. I was like Beaver stuffing food in his face after June Cleaver asks, "Anyone know what happened to my new crystal bowl?" Pan to the Beave picturing his worm collection enjoying their beautiful new crystal home.

I felt bad, but what could I do? And really, how would it have looked to turn myself in? That morning it had all seemed very sensible and aboveboard, but in hindsight it made me look like quite the deviant. Like I was one bad decision away from unbridled bestiality.

I just didn't get it. Why would a dog lick my foot for twenty minutes if it was making him sick? I filed away this new revelation along with the results of my doing-whatever-I-felt-like experiment from college. I knew there was an intelligence, an order, a force, if you will, to nature and the universe, but I just didn't have it all figured out yet.

Thankfully, Rocky was fine by the evening, back to his old self, prancing around the apartment, alternating between naps on the couch, sips of water from his bowl, and a quick hump or two on his female counterpart, Twinkie.

So back to High Point, North Carolina, where on that chilly and rainy day, I feared cat ass and checked the trusty gym directory for the nearest location. Twenty minutes later I arrived at the only reciprocal gym in town and was surprised to find that there was no aerobics room and no mats for stretching whatsoever. I was disappointed but vaguely remembered that on the way I had passed a massage center. I figured, "Wow, a massage center, they've got to have a yoga space. Maybe I can even catch a class." So I retraced my path and found the spot. It was called Ruby's Massage.

The front door did not open, so I knocked. A woman opened the door, with the chain still on, and peeked out at me. "Yes, can I help you?"

"Um, do you have a yoga space I can use?"

She must have thought me a loon, or maybe she thought, "Hmm, the yoga treatment. Well, I'd need the trampoline, an initiation paddle, three strap restraints, and a few sticky mats." Either way, all she said was, "No, but we do offer massage."

I've always considered massage to be like passive yoga — you get all the same benefits but without any of the hard work. I figure that's why you pay for it. So I was intrigued.

"How much?" I asked.

"Thirty for a half-hour, sixty for an hour."

"Fair prices," I thought.

"And it's topless," she added.

"No problem," I said. "At Kripalu I'm totally naked when I get a massage."

She nodded but seemed perplexed.

Now, I'm not sure at what point in the above dialogue you caught on, but I was still naively in the dark. Up until then, the only massages I had received were in the small offices of licensed massage therapists at gyms or at Kripalu. When I met up with Zach later that day, he said I should have been tipped off by the fact that the place was called Ruby's Massage and certainly by the fact that Ruby opened the door with the chain still on, as if I was querying at a 1920s speakeasy. But I'm proud to say that in my quest for yoga I was in some sort of purist, naive state, totally unaware that this sort of thing even existed and totally oblivious to where I was headed.

I began to clue in moments later, though, when she opened the door to let me in and I took in my surroundings. Slowly it hit me: "Hmm, red-velvet wallpaper," "Hmm, matching red-velvet lampshades." I don't know if movies imitate real life or if real life imitates movies, but it seemed that I was upstairs at an Old West saloon, right out of Clint Eastwood's *Unforgiven*. Finally Ruby brought me into a massage room that confirmed any lingering doubts I might have had. There was no massage table, only a bed — red velvet.

At Kripalu the massage therapist leaves the room while you undress to your own level of comfort and slide under the generous, thick massage table sheet. This bed had no top sheet, only a very bare, red-velvet, fitted sheet.

Ruby told me to undress but did not leave the room. In fact, she was busy running my credit card as I undressed right there in front of her. She ignored me as though I were browsing for shoes, except when the credit card slip was ready and I think she actually handed it to me to sign while my pants were still on one leg. She was either used to all this and oblivious to my discomfort, or she actually enjoyed the power. She told me to lie facedown on the bed. I did as I was told. She was a bit dominant, really, but thankfully that is *not* where this story is headed.

Ruby got on top of me and started massaging my back and shoulders while gyrating on my butt. I was pretty uncomfortable, and the massage was really not very good. Clinging to a false reality, I asked, "Where did you study massage?" She named some school I had never heard of. At least she was playing along.

"You're not a regular massage therapist," I added brilliantly.

"Turn over," she instructed.

I knew a turnover would bring this to a whole new level of vulnerability, and I was nervous. "Fearless, honest, relaxed," I thought, and I turned over.

The technical massage term for covering a client is *draping*. Ruby "draped" me in a washcloth. She sat right on the cloth and continued the massage. And that's when the topless promise kicked in. This was indeed a topless massage. Ruby flicked some shoulder clips and her shirt dropped off, leaving her business to mostly sag and sometimes bounce around as she *effleuraged* my pecs and shoulders.

Maybe I should have relaxed and enjoyed it, but that was not in my nature. I felt bad that she was doing this for a living, I was not attracted to her, and I'd always been a bit of a bacteriaphobe — so I was very busy at failing to keep my mind from considering the red-velvet fitted sheet on which I lay naked. I imagined the black light from *CSI* or *Basic Instinct* illuminating all the hidden stains.

Ruby woke me from these disturbed musings with the obvious question (since, really, why else would anyone be there?), "Would you like any special services?"

There I was, stark naked, nauseated, and lying on this prostitute's red-velvet bed in the middle of the day, when eighteen minutes earlier I had been looking for a yoga space. At this point "fearless, honest, relaxed" threatened to be my undoing, like saying "yes" was for Jim Carrey's character in *Yes Man*. Terrified of her response, I gulped, steadied myself, and squeaked out, "What kind of special services?"

Ruby's answer still makes me cringe; speaking in an emotionally detached way about sex makes me very uncomfortable, like hearing nails on a chalkboard. So when she let me know, "Hand release $30, oral release $60," I could have vomited on the spot.

I don't know why, probably too many episodes of *Law and Order*, but I said, "How do you know I'm not a cop?"

"You're no cop," was all she said. She was right. The thin, bearded hippie on her red-velvet bed didn't look much like a police officer. I'd have to be full-tilt Donnie Brasco — deep undercover, after months of character development, and I guess she knew that her small operation would not merit such a masterful sting.

I did not enjoy my time at Ruby's. Afterward I headed straight back to the gym and scrubbed like Meryl Streep in *Silkwood* after the plutonium accident.

I can tell you that this experience certainly did not cheapen my respect for sex or my esteem for monogamous relationships. On the contrary, it cemented the realization that, for me, sex without emotion, or at least without mutual attraction, would be empty and depressing and depleting.

When I later got home from the trip and told Yolanthe of my escapades at Ruby's, she shared that one of the best orgasms of her life had been at the skilled hands of such a masseuse. Her story was a bit more romantic, perhaps — on the ocean in Mexico in the 1970s. And she was certainly a bit more free-spirited than I. Yolanthe assumed the orgasm was part of the package at the spa. That's just how Yolanthe rolled, to assume an orgasm came with the deal. It made me wonder if my Victorian discomfort had infected what could have been a more enjoyable and less regrettably guilt-ridden and disturbing affair.

After my post-Ruby's scrub-down, I went to meet Zach at one of the many buffet restaurants that bespeckle the South. As a northerner, I was intrigued by these buffets. I find them a bit of a paradox, really. Each individual dish offered at the buffet is irredeemably vile, and yet the sheer variety of foods seems to make up for their insipid flavor. It's as though each dish holds a new potential for enjoyment, or maybe the magnitude of offerings is just a hoot in and of itself. I suppose it's archetypically American — lots and lots of choices and lots and lots of food and lots and lots of people slopping it down.

Zach was eager to tell me about his adventures, benign and pedestrian, of course, as they stood in comparison to mine. I let him talk first, which I knew would add to the drama when I finally laid it on him, like when someone natters on for thirty minutes about window treatments before a friend finally drops the "I'm pregnant" bombshell.

Zach had previously lived for two years in High Point, so his first response was, "Jeez, Leaf, did anyone see you pull in? People around here know that van belongs to me." And then his second response was, "*How* could you not know?"

I told him the whole story. He thought it was absolutely terrific and enjoyed every single minute of it. But I felt pretty sullied, and it took me a day or two to fully recover. Perhaps, though, I was a man now, at least in my ability to recognize a whorehouse when I saw one, or maybe in my new, fuller appreciation of a loving relationship.

Chapter 10

Jerry Garcia

Once in a while you get shown the light
in the strangest of places if you look at it right.
— JERRY GARCIA and ROBERT HUNTER, "Scarlet Begonias"

Apart from the Ruby business, I had a great time in High Point. We were staying with Howard and Alexandra, and they were pretty free. Well, sort of free. Howard smoked a fair bit of pot, which cloaked his neurotic side and made him *seem* free. He was a pretty typical pot smoker: a nervous guy, uncomfortable in his own skin, and uncomfortable in his relationships. He had become comfortable with his wife, Alexandra, and a lot of pot smokers are like that, uncomfortable with people in general but invested in one person with whom they can relax and be themselves. Usually it's a partner, but there are lots of platonic examples too, such as Beavis and Butthead and *Superbad*'s Seth and Evan.

Howard smoked to make the rest of the day more comfortable. It took the edge off work for him. It took the edge off interacting with others. It took the edge off his nerves and his physical tension. He'd actually have done well with some yoga instead. Yoga has the same perks but without the side effects, and it's cheaper.

In my observation, using pot the way that Howard did works for a time, but eventually, after a decade or so, leaves a person very anxious or even with an anxiety disorder. I'm not sure if the pot affects a person's nerves and brain chemistry over time. More likely it merely covers but does not actually soothe the nervousness and anxiety, which build up and then overflow or explode later. Pot prevents a person from dealing with his discomfort, which without the pot, he would have been forced to address. Without the pot, he would have more motivation to express his feelings, to develop communication skills, to exercise to relieve the stress, or even to pursue psychotherapy for the anxiety.

I know marijuana is used regularly in certain cultures without causing mass anxiety disorder, but I'm just saying that here in the United States, most of the folks whom I've seen use pot every day for an extended period as a way to calm their nerves or ease the tension they feel when interacting with others eventually get very anxious.

It might not surprise you that Howard and Alexandra were former Deadheads. They were not actually former; in fact, they were still quite active, but now they had jobs and could not tour with the Grateful Dead as they used to. Before buying their apartment, Howard and Alexandra were full-on, the kind of folks who go on tour selling peanut-butter-and-jelly sandwiches in the parking lot to pay for traveling expenses. They were the kind of hippies you see walking around the parking lot in quilted shirts with a finger in the air "looking for a miracle." When we were visiting, the Dead were actually coming through nearby Charlotte, North Carolina, so Howard and Alexandra got tickets for us all.

I had been to a Dead show one other time, four years earlier, but that was a very different time. That was in 1991, during the summer between my sophomore and junior years of college. I had just recovered from mono, which had caused me to leave Georgetown two weeks early. I went to the concert with my buddy Beard and his friend Beard Beard.

It was a very hot day at the Meadowlands in East Rutherford, New Jersey. It was so hot and sunny that Beard Beard had gotten a sunburn on his arm while resting it out his open window as he drove to the concert. Driving to the Meadowlands stadium in New Jersey was a surreal experience to begin with. Driving the long, winding approach to the complex, one grasps the shadow of what must once have been there, of the ecological melting pot robust with bird, fish, and plant species. But instead you now have the clear sense that if your car broke down and you had to walk to the stadium, and if you, God forbid, made the brash and imprudent decision to cut across the swamp, you'd either get eaten by a nuclear-enhanced crocodile or turned into the Joker from *Batman*.

In fact, that sense of foreboding is in no way misplaced. The Meadowlands has seen decades of abuse from every variety of hazardous waste dumping. After World War II, ships returning home from London even dumped actual war rubble from the Battle of Britain. They had been using the debris as ballast and then ditched it in the Meadowlands. So the vague sense of the Meadowlands as a war zone is totally justified.

So Beard, Beard Beard, and I had driven the distance, waited in traffic, and found a parking spot among the carnival that was a Dead show parking lot. It was like Cirque du Soleil or a scene out of an art house movie. There were stilt walkers, dazzling displays of colorful clothing, and people selling hits of nitro (laughing gas) out of giant balloons.

Since I was recovering from mono, I did not share the gallon jug of water that my friends were passing around. And later I lost them in the swaying mass of Deadheads doing their distinctive Deadhead dance. I knew that I was feeling a bit fatigued from the mono, but I didn't realize that the heat and lack of water were taking a toll on me.

About halfway into the concert I nearly passed out from dehydration. I hobbled my way over to the concession stand to get some water, then sank down in the shade on the cool concrete to rest and drink. I must have looked quite a sight, since more than one person walked by and with earnest compassion said things like, "Bad trip, dude?" "Can I get you anything?" and "It'll be all right. Process through it, man."

Four years later, I was more mature, it was not 98 degrees, and I had my own bottle of water. Or perhaps the main difference was my guides. Howard and Alexandra called Zach and me virgins, meaning it was our first show (or second, in my case), and they guided us with tenderness and care. Actually, it was more Alexandra who guided us. Howard toked up and took off. For Alexandra, going to a Dead show was like attending church. It was a place to pray, find inspiration, and connect with spirit.

Alexandra believed that at each show she had to find her right place, her power spot, in the venue. She led us from section to section within the arena. A stadium in full Dead-show mode is quite a scene, even more so than the circus of the parking lot. It's a traveling Woodstock. It's *Alice in Wonderland*, Spanish carnival, and a concert of medieval minstrels all mixed together. And it definitely required multiple repetitions of "Fearless, honest, relaxed" as well as "When in Rome" for me to get comfortable.

Alexandra led us to a large open space, and we danced in a swirling mass of tie-dyed Deadhead dervishes. I really let loose with the dancing, and since admittedly I'm not the most natural dancer, Alexandra had to reposition me more than once to prevent me from knocking people over as I noodled my body with the music.

Alexandra kept moving us to a new part of the arena, and I began to get annoyed. Each time I settled into a place, she'd move us, looking for her right spot. At one point we were sitting on the bleachers way up high and very far from the stage. We were sitting and watching and listening. Since I didn't know most of the words, I was singing along to each song's chorus as best I could. "So many roads, so many roads / Mountain high, river wide / So many roads to ride."

Eventually I stopped singing and surrendered to *feeling* the music. I closed my eyes as my body swayed on the bleacher seat. I was drawn further in and began focusing singly on feeling the music vibrating in my body. My insides began to stir as the music awoke an energy within me. The energy built and built. My body started pulsating. And then, no lie, I saw a green light travel directly from my chest through the air across the stadium and right into Jerry Garcia's guitar. I was plugged in.

Then the green light began to push me back. I had to hook my toes under the bleacher to keep from being knocked over. I began chanting "om" like I did in yoga class. Tears streamed down my cheeks. I was filled with exultation. I was exploding with bliss and energy. I thought that I was literally going to have an orgasm (since I had no other experience with which to compare or interpret my current sensations).

I almost leaned over to tell Alexandra of my ecstasy. I'm glad I didn't, because "I think I might orgasm" is what I would have said, and even in full Dead-show regalia, I'm not sure it's biblically legal to say that to a married woman.

A few moments later, Alexandra tugged on my sleeve and pulled me up from my reverie. She was my guide, and I obediently followed. I assumed she knew exactly what I was experiencing and was leading me to a secret meeting of those who were plugged in, a special gathering of Jerry's chosen few who "got it" and received the blessing of his green light.

Unfortunately, however, Alexandra was just moving us again to find her right spot. Upon being moved, I came down from my exultation. I craved the high and spent the rest of the show, unsuccessfully, trying to recapture the feeling.

I swear to you that (as far as I know) I had taken no acid or mushrooms or psychedelic drugs of any kind. Perhaps, in the Lewis Carroll novel that is a Grateful Dead show, these substances are unnecessary. Perhaps the swirling energy of the place, fueled by the free-spiritedness of the Deadheads, by the sound and poetry of the music, and presumably by Jerry himself, was enough to bring about this transcendence.

And at that time I had not yet learned about the chakras (energy centers in the body), and I didn't know that the heart chakra, located, of course, in the chest, is associated with the color green. I had also never heard stories of high-energy states that practitioners sometimes experience in the presence of a guru or master. Usually the experience involves an awakening of energy that brings bliss, tears, and exultation.

The day after the show, I felt transformed. I was going to tour with the Dead and bathe in Jerry's green light. I had found my home and my new style of yoga. It was called the Grateful Dead.

Two things happened to change that. First, I settled back into my life and my yoga practice, and a life on the road with the Grateful Dead did not seem as alluring. And second, the show that I saw in Charlotte, North Carolina, in March 1995 with my friends, was part of the first tour in which the Dead played the song "Unbroken Chain." When the song began, all the joyous Deadheads in their sleeveless quilted shirts stopped swaying and started booing. I turned to Alexandra for an explanation. She was staring at the stage, openmouthed, looking appalled and angry. She told me that the Dead had never, ever played "Unbroken Chain" at a concert, and she told me that according to the legend, when they played it, it would signal the end of their days of touring.

Sure enough, this legend proved to be correct. The Grateful Dead released "Unbroken Chain" on their album *Grateful Dead from the Mars Hotel* in 1974 and had not played the song live in concert in the twenty-one years since its release. I don't know what Jerry, Phil, and Bob were thinking when they segued into that song that day in Charlotte, but five months later, on August 9, 1995, the world lost Jerry Garcia to a heart attack.

I was at Kripalu when I heard the news. I was very sad to hear it. I had not taken up residence on a VW bus selling peanut-butter-and-jelly sandwiches, but I understood that Jerry Garcia was indeed a channel for some sort of ecstatic force of love, and I knew that his presence would be dearly missed.

Chapter 11

Flatulence

This one is a bit embarrassing.

You're probably thinking, "But, Brian, you have admitted to seeing a hooker; what's more embarrassing than that?" True enough. But what was even more embarrassing than accidentally seeing a prostitute (and I must firmly remind you that my visit was entirely accidental) was uncontrollable flatulence.

I had determined that my role as a yogi-hippie required vegetarianism. People don't realize that being a vegetarian, or at least doing it right — getting enough protein and eating enough fresh vegetables — is pretty difficult, especially on the road, as in the terrific scene in *Everything Is Illuminated* when Elijah Wood's character is traveling in Eastern Europe. At a Ukrainian restaurant he informs the waitress that's he's a vegetarian and can't eat kielbasa. She looks him up and down like he's deranged (much like Ricky's mom often eyeballed me), humphs, and returns with one peeled boiled potato.

Being a vegetarian on the road in 1995, especially in the breadbasket of the Great Plains or in the Deep South, was pretty similar. Often, my meal consisted of peanut butter and bananas, or in a restaurant, of iceberg lettuce and three-bean salad. Keep in mind that Zach and I were on a budget.

One time I actually opened a can of cold vegetarian chili at a rest stop and ate it right out of the can. That's when things went south. Unless you have a belly of steel, I do not recommend eating cold veggie chili right out of the can on a cold, damp morning. Especially because the TVP (textured vegetable protean) in veggie chili makes it much harder to digest than ordinary meat chili. I'm not sure that TVP was initially intended as a human comestible. It's like one of those over-the-counter drugs originally invented for use as an adhesive, giant panda aphrodisiac, or horse tranquilizer.

First I tried to grin and bear it. But eventually, in Hot Springs, Arkansas, after a few weeks on the road, I was desperate. I even responded to an annoying chain letter that threatened me harm were I not to pass it along. I had been ignoring the letter and thought perhaps it was the secret, pernicious cause of my intestinal discomfort. When replying to that letter didn't work, I broke down and decided to turn to Western medicine for help.

I waited in the Hot Springs walk-in clinic and filled out the paperwork:

Name: *Brian Leaf*

Reason for visit: *Really bad gas*

The clinic was the sort of place that people come to for urgent, acute medical problems, like knife wounds and dog bites. I was there because of gas and because I was a thousand miles from my primary care physician.

Finally a nurse called my name and walked me to an examining room. When the doctor, accustomed to lacerations and bloody coughs, came in, he thought a buddy was playing a joke on him when I presented with, basically, stinky farts. He occasionally peeked at the door, waiting, I think, for a coworker or even Ashton Kutcher to pop out. He listened suspiciously. Our conversation went something like this:

"What can I do for you (*Yankee scum*)?"

"Ah, I'm having stomach trouble."

"Pains?"

"Uh, no, um, smelly gas. (*Should I show him? I can easily produce on cue, right here and now.*)"

"Aha...and how long have you had this, ah...problem?"

"Several weeks."

At this point, he checks the door, maybe for Allen Funt, or maybe because he's anxious to get back to the patient in room 3 who's bleeding out from a knife wound.

"Um, I don't think I can help you with that. Have you tried Gas-X?"

I explain to him that I had colitis and that my previous doctor had given me stomach relaxers for similar symptoms a few years earlier.

When speaking to this very kindly Arkansas doctor in 1995, I did not yet realize that twenty years of stored anxiety and repressed anger was living in my colon, weakening my digestion, and, after being awoken in Janice's yoga class, readying itself for a cathartic release. But that's probably just as well, for his sake and mine, since he was already sweating like a pig, vexed by my farts, and worried about being caught on TV in a prank.

I'm also not surprised that the doctor didn't pick up on the immediate, short-term cause of my problem. Not too many people in Arkansas eat TVP, and I suspect consuming veggie chili in certain counties of the South might be punishable by public flogging. If nothing else, it is a blasphemous sacrilege, a direct offense against great-grandma Ed's award-winning recipe. The only crime more notoriously villainous is using soymilk in corn bread.

Although the doctor could provide little insight into my problem, I did succeed in convincing him to prescribe the stomach relaxers. I filled his prescription at a local pharmacy, and the meds helped a lot. It was not until Chicago, several weeks later, however, when I picked up a book on Ayurveda, that I got some deeper answers.

Ayurveda is a five-thousand-year-old holistic medical system from India, often called the sister science of yoga, and it is brilliant. According to Ayurveda, there are different types of people, and these different types have different needs. For example, while spinach indisputably contains abundant vitamins and minerals, some people digest it well and integrate its nutrition, while others don't, and the nutrition is lost on them.

Ayurveda not only predicts who will and will not easily digest spinach but also offers ways of making it more digestible for each constitutional type — cook it, eat it raw, use oil, don't use oil, make it spicy, keep it mild.

I'm not sure why the West skipped over this system. It makes perfect sense. How crazy is it to assume that everyone has exactly the same needs and benefits from the same foods? As one of the most famous Ayurvedic physicians, Deepak Chopra, teaches, a roller coaster causes an endorphin reaction in some people worth $10,000 of medication, and it makes others sick.

Best of all, Ayurveda, whose practitioners have observed people for thousands of years, has a way of telling which type of person you are and therefore which foods to eat, which exercises to use, and even at which jobs you'll thrive.

I discovered that types like me, called *vata*, do better with warm, cooked food, and that beans and soy products might be a bit tough on my belly. The book very nearly described the worst possible meal for a *vata* person as cold TVP veggie chili right out of the can at a rest stop on a cool, wet North Carolina morning.

Chapter 12

The Yamas and Niyamas

Yama and *niyama* are the seeds of yoga.

— SWAMI KRIPALU

Zach and I had nowhere in particular to go and all the time in the world to get there. We'd pull into a town, Zach would find a café or bookstore, and I'd find the yoga classes. I became a master at finding yoga in a new town. (So far I had taken Iyengar, Integral, Ananda, and Ashtanga classes but had yet to fall in love again.) Too bad there was no game show that pitted contestants against one another: the first to find the yoga classes wins. I could do it in, like, three minutes flat. The best bet was to hit the health food store and check the bulletin board. In the absence of a health food store, I'd check the public library board. Sometimes the classes were even held right in the library basement.

Time on our trip moved at a different pace, the way time moves on a camping trip. At home on a Tuesday morning, when you're running late for work, chores such as brushing teeth and cooking breakfast can become to-dos, to be checked off before the actual focus of the morning. But when traveling or camping, brushing teeth, cooking breakfast, and having a stroll *are* the morning's activity.

Zach and I would wake up and then look for a place to wash.

We'd have breakfast and then have a hike or find a tea shop and play chess with the locals. I discovered that the homeless are uncanny chess players.

At night, when we weren't staying on the sofas of the members of Zach's singing group, we'd look for a good place to park and sleep.

Out in the countryside or in state parks I felt very comfortable in the van at night. I loved hearing the spring peepers and seeing the stars and moon through the window. But sleeping in cities presented different sights and sounds, and sleeping in the van parallel parked on city streets scared me. So we hatched a plan to park and sleep in hotel parking lots. The parking lots were patrolled and felt much safer than the street.

We also soon discovered that as long as we pretended to look like we belonged, we could use a hotel's facilities — brush our teeth in the bathroom, have a leisurely dip in the pool, even eat the continental breakfast spread. Zach was a fan of the cheese Danishes, and I enjoyed the bagels and instant hot oatmeal packets. We were living large for free.

This was working out very well for us. Sadly, it soon became clear that it was not working out so well for the hotels. The night-time patrols were there not just to keep the parked cars safe but to keep squatters like us off the premises.

One night, at a four-star hotel in San Diego, a group of night patrols deemed the van suspicious. We awoke to flashlights and batons tapping at the glass of the windows.

Thankfully, the back windows of the van were tinted, and we had also rigged drapes, so they couldn't see in. Still, I was terrified and would have turned us in to the mercy of the law right then and there. But Zach, always a cooler customer than I, shushed me. He was like Russell Crowe in *Gladiator* (or was it Mel Gibson in *Brave-heart?*): "Wait…wait…wait…*now!*" and as soon as the patrollers walked off to consult the hotel manager or call the police, he jumped up from lying on his back on the futon to sitting in the driver's seat, started the van, and screeched off, all in a single motion. It was impressive.

Another time at a Comfort Inn in Texas, I was brushing my teeth in the bathroom when a very menacing-looking security guard, who had probably received a tip, came in and brusquely escorted me off the premises with many belligerent promises if I were to return. He said he never forgot a face. I felt like Chris McCandless, caught by railroad security for tramping on freight cars.

This lifestyle was scary but also educational and a bit exhilarating. When my family traveled when I was a kid, we had always been part of the paying clientele, enjoying the hotel facilities and being treated by hotel staff as though we owned the place. It was interesting and educational to be on the other side. There's nothing like wearing the other shoe to build some compassion.

The breakfasts were, of course, meant for paying hotel guests, not for wandering hippies who sleep covertly in the parking lot. I'm not sure how all this had thus far escaped the test of my travel mantra: "fearless, *honest*, relaxed."

But then one day, as I entered a Marriott in Denver, Colorado, heading for the breakfast spread, I realized that my shoulders were a bit hunched and that, literally and figuratively, I was looking over my shoulder, wary of a wise security guard or front-desk clerk who might catch on. Quite a bit of my concentration was devoted to watching for patrols and worrying about getting caught.

J. R. R. Tolkien, when he wrote *The Lord of the Rings* trilogy, understood this phenomenon in the character of Gollum. Gollum killed his friend to steal the ring, and he becomes consumed and contorted by remorse. He turns from a hobbit, like Bilbo and Frodo, into a hunched, demented creature, coveting the ring and looking over his shoulder for would-be hijackers. I was turning into Gollum for my "precious" hotel bagels and oatmeal.

I realized that to dedicate myself fully to yoga and the pursuit of liberation, I would need all my energy available to me, not frittered away watching for the law. I finally understood why nonstealing might be an important precept for a yogi.

All religions have these rules of behavior: the Judeo-Christian Ten Commandments, the Yogic *yamas* and *niyamas*, the Buddhist precepts, the Islamic moral codes, and so on. Perhaps the rules are designed to keep order in society. You can't just sleep with your neighbor when you feel the urge, and you can't just nick a cheese Danish from a hotel when you feel a bit peckish.

Perhaps these rules are the will of God, there to help you secure your place in heaven. And perhaps they are there to help seekers manage their energy, to channel maximum vitality to the pursuit of freedom.

In Hebrew school as a child, studying for my bar mitzvah, I learned the Ten Commandments. And from yoga classes and books, I learned the *yamas* and *niyamas*. But this hotel experience opened my eyes and heart to their purpose for me.

I think a person who is tuned in to her intuition and heart would ultimately not need rules; she would act morally. It would simply feel bad to lie, steal, or harm others. Put another way, if my consciousness were clear, I'd see the correct choices in front of me, and they would be the most appealing options.

But in the process of conducting psychospiritual experiments, in the process of trying out new ways of being and of cultivating intuition and heart, the rules are essential. At first, judgment is clouded. As I learned from my college experiment of doing only what I wanted, until intuition is strengthened, there must be will and adherence to plans and rules. Only after lots of self-exploration and experimentation and growth would what I want be clean and just, a direct extension of my heart, a flowing act of energy made manifest. But at first I needed the rules. Otherwise, I could end up three weeks later in vomit-stained clothes, with a twisted ankle, and behind on three weeks of homework.

Recall from the last chapter that, according to Ayurveda, there are different types of people, and these different types have different needs. Here too, after lots of self-exploration and experimentation and healthy living, one's needs would become intuitively clear — one's urges would perfectly match his best interests. But at first, he would need to follow dietary guidelines and lifestyle suggestions.

Sometimes I like to do an experiment: I pick one *yama* or *niyama* and follow it "religiously" for a week. This works because, as Swami Kripalu says, the *yamas* and *niyamas* are like beads on a necklace — if you pick up one, they all follow along. Actually, he said it a bit more poetically: "By firmly grasping the flower of a single virtue, a person can lift the entire garland of *yama* and *niyama*." In other words, dedicated practice of any one of the *yamas* or *niyamas* will result in cultivation of them all.

For example, if you follow nonharming, you can't lie to a friend because at some level the lie will harm her. Swami Kripalu also meant that practicing any one of the rules builds consciousness. And increased consciousness will make a person desire the comfort, peace, and joy afforded by adherence to all the rules.

Try this. Pick one *yama* or *niyama* to follow for the next week, and see how you feel. Let us know how it goes at www.Misadventures -of-a-Yogi.com.

Here, then, without further ado, are the ten yogic *yamas* and *niyamas*:

nonviolence (*ahimsa*)
truthfulness (*satya*)
nonstealing (*asteya*)
moderation (*brahmacharya*)

noncovetousness (*aparigraha*)
purity, cleanliness (*shaucha*)
contentment, gratitude (*santosha*)
discipline, purpose (*tapas*)
self-observation, reflection (*swadhyaya*)
meditation on the divine (*Ishvara-pranidhana*)

And with these *yamas* and *niyamas* in mind, let's revisit our second Key to Happiness:

Follow your heart.

Ground rules such as the *yamas* and *niyamas* are critical in this process. If an urge violates a rule, you must ignore it. If you feel like starting a business by selling your younger brother into servitude, ehhhnnt, no sale. If you want to leave your spouse and fourteen children for a new life with your twenty-three-year-old Zumba instructor, that's probably a misinterpretation of following bliss. This is not libido or ego or thrill we're talking about, and the *yamas* and *niyamas* help clarify that. Following your heart should not involve stealing, lying, or hurting. If it does, it's probably fear, insecurity, or ego masquerading as heart. You can't achieve true freedom, heart, or bliss on the backs of others. Noam Chomsky will tell you that.

Unfortunately, my new appreciation for the *yamas* and *niyamas* meant sacrificing my free, basically stolen, morning bagels and oatmeal.

But fortunately, oatmeal at most diners across the country rang in under two bucks, and eating oatmeal without looking over my shoulder both relaxed my stomach and made the oats a whole lot tastier.

Chapter 13

Jemez

Zach and I discovered that if someone, say, Zach's uncle, or even our idol, Zach's sociology professor, fearless-honest-and-relaxed Richard, recommended visiting a certain town or landmark because he had had a memorable adventure there, that did not necessarily mean that we would as well. We discovered that a place would not, on its own, determine the depth of our adventure.

Our experience of a town was partly determined by the mood we were in when we arrived. Were we open to the place and its adventure, or were we tired and closed off, ready to zone out and rest?

Even more so, though, the depth of our adventure was determined by the people we met. Our guidebooks were informative and interesting, and helped us find high-quality cheap food and odd roadside attractions, such as a one-hundred-year-old fruitcake in Hurricane, Utah, and the little rock that gives the capital of Arkansas its name. But in Hot Springs, Arkansas, when John and Annie Dicksie took us prospecting in the Ouachita Mountains for quartz crystals and sent us away with a bottle of fresh honey from their neighbor's bees, now, that was a high.

So by the time we got to New Mexico we understood this dynamic well, and as soon as we pulled into Albuquerque, we stopped a few college students and asked them what to do in town. Sometimes when we asked this question, the answer was as simple as a bar with good music, sometimes it was a poetry slam that evening, sometimes it was a pick-up soccer game or a favorite hiking spot, but that day in Albuquerque we hit the jackpot. The students told us of a hot springs deep in the woods, and they gave us directions.

We were to drive west on Route 4 and after about thirty minutes look for a pull-off on the right. We were to park, walk on a log to cross a river, and then hike up the mountain, keeping an eye out for trickling water. "Once you spot the trickling water," they said, "follow it up the mountain, and you'll find the hot springs."

We headed west on 4 but couldn't find the parking lot. We pulled into a Zen monastery to ask directions from a monk in full Zen getup. He looked just like John C. Reilly in Adam Sandler's *Anger Management*. Thankfully he was not under a vow of silence.

The monk told us that we were looking for Jemez Hot Springs and that we had not actually missed the pull-off. We were only minutes away. We found the lot, parked the car, crossed the log, and hiked up the mountain, watching for trickling water. We caught a glimpse of a trickle and followed it up. Up and up and up, and then suddenly right over a ridge, there we were.

I know I like to paint myself as a hippie on the road, but inside I was still the white-shirt-and-khaki-pants-wearing Georgetown business school grad from suburban New Jersey, so I was surprised by the wildness of the terrain out west. It made New Jersey seem like a manicured theme park governed by safety regulations.

A place like Jemez Hot Springs in New Jersey would have guardrails, handrails, and antiskid stairways. There would be a fee for parking and a chair lift so that you could enjoy the springs without the hike. In New Jersey, this might have been called Bank of America Hot Springs.

But in Jemez, there were no guardrails, no park ranger, no pay phones, no advertisements, no hot dog stands, and no carefully chosen Kodak-sponsored photo-op stations. Even relaxed by yoga, touched by Jerry Garcia, and made a man by Ruby, I was completely unprepared for the scene when we arrived at the springs.

You know the phenomenon from hiking: you're climbing a ridge when suddenly new scenery pops right out from behind a large tree as if from nowhere. Well, one minute we were alone following the trickle, and the next we were in *The Doors* movie.

There were three pools of different temperatures. Each pool, about the size of a large Jacuzzi, was lined with smooth stones and earth and moss and had been there for who knows how long. The highest pool was fed by the spring and was the hottest. Water poured out of the highest into two successive pools, each slightly cooler than the previous.

There were perhaps ten naked people in and around the tubs soaking, relaxing, and drying in the sun. There was even a Native American man with a long ponytail, stark naked and covered in mud, who was lying spread-eagled on the ground, basking in the sun. I think he was asleep.

This was all too much for us, so we just nodded "hello" casually and kept walking as though we were accustomed to this sort of thing and were just passing through.

Finally, after another quarter mile or so up the mountain, Zach stopped and said, "This is crazy. Why are we afraid? Let's just do it," and he stripped off his pants and started trotting down to the springs.

There's something so comical and sweet about a person clothed only above the waist, like a toddler run off from the potty without a fresh diaper. I'd say it's more vulnerable than being fully naked.

At least then you're sending a clear, unified message that says, "I'm free, as nature made me!" but being exposed only down below highlights the contrast between clothed and naked and says, "I have a nay-ked tu-shie!"

So there was Zach trotting down the hill, UNC sweatshirt on, and nothing else.

I followed behind.

Zach arrived at the tubs, finished stripping, and climbed in.

"Good for him," I thought.

I was a bit jealous of his aplomb, and I wasn't quite ready to strip and hop in, so I chatted with some folks on the side for a while.

There were several different groups at the springs. There was a VW busload of folks on a Phish tour who were living at the springs while the band took a break from touring. There were a few (very attractive and naked) women in their twenties from a nearby naturopathic medical college, and then there was the Indian who no one actually knew or had seen move, I think. The Phish folks invited us to visit their campsite that night for a bonfire.

After a while and a few resolute repetitions of "fearless, honest, relaxed," I disrobed and slid in.

The water and the scene were completely liberating. There're no two ways about it; being naked is freeing. Being naked is also vulnerable, but that's part of the liberation — being less guarded. I was naked in a natural hot spring in the earth, on a mountain surrounded by Phishheads, naturopathic medical students, and a mysterious Indian. The trees were vibrantly green and the birds were brilliant blue.

I'd like to say that I was so mature that I wasn't thinking, "Boobies!" That the Steve Stifler part of my brain had been left at the New Jersey state line. But there I was naked with these amazing naturopathic medical school women, whom I would have been enamored of even clothed. So *American Pie* was in full effect. At first. And then

I settled in and got comfortable and primal and got into the vibe of the group. Seinfeld said that people will fantasize about whatever others have to cover up. If women were required to cover their elbows, men would walk around all day saying, "Did you see the elbows on that one?"

Before long, I was just hanging out with other souls, enjoying being part of nature together on a beautiful, sparkling day.

The Jemez regulars told us that because we were in a state park, we could park overnight in the pull-off where we had left our van. So we hiked down, got our gear, and returned to set up camp.

That night we joined the Phishies for their bonfire. I got in a deep conversation with two dreadlocked women about Jerry Garcia and his green light. They appreciated my experience but were eager to convert me to worshipping, instead, at the altar of Trey Anastasio, Mike Gordon, Jon Fishman, and Page McConnell. I thought I had a chance with one of the women, but then I got really cold and had to head back to my tent. Stumbling over rocks and roots and weaving through trees, I was terrified that I'd get lost in the pitch-black.

I found my tent and crawled in. When I woke up in the morning, I did some lovely yoga. On my way I passed the springs, and two of the Phishies, I'd say the two leaders of their clan, were in the coolest spring. I thought they were just hugging, so I said, "Hello." It was the polite thing to do. But then I realized it was a rhythmically moving hug. I can't recall, but I don't think they said "Hi" back.

After I finished yoga, I settled into the hottest tub for a soak. I even did some gentle *pranayama* (yogic breathing) and chanting in the tub.

Chapter 14

White Sands

There are three ways to be in the world:
1. To believe that we are each alone and separate from one another.
2. To realize that we are all connected.
And 3. To realize that we are all one.

— RAM DASS, lecture in Northampton, Massachusetts, 2003

Zach and I had stumbled onto paradise. You'd think that nothing could have pulled us away from this Eden. But I started having an urge, like an itch that burns, to return to White Sands, New Mexico. Zach and I had been there two days earlier, but we had arrived only a few minutes before the park closed, so we snapped a few photos and then hit the road.

White Sands is a giant white dune in the middle of southern New Mexico. The area was created 100 million years ago when a sea evaporated and left behind mineral deposits of white gypsum. Over millions of years the deposits eroded into fine white sand crystals. Unlike the quartz-based sand that you find in deserts and at the beach, this white gypsum sand stays cool in the sun. That means that even on a scorching New Mexico day, you can walk barefoot on the soothing, white sand.

White Sands has the dubious distinction of being the testing site for the first atom bomb in 1945. Think about the destruction and violence of that fact. It's staggering. And this darkness is in stark and shocking contrast to the very spiritual feel of the national monument portion, which has a very vital feel, like the red rock vortexes of new age Sedona, Arizona.

As Zach and I traveled, I practiced yoga and meditation in each of the areas we trekked through. Part of my travelogue was a mental note of my yoga experiences, of how yoga felt in each place. Imagine practicing in bustling New York City, in a Victorian on Cape Cod, on a farm in rural Wisconsin, at an ashram in California, and in a white-sand desert, and you'll see what I mean. So when we were in White Sands, I felt the urge to practice yoga there, but because we were in a rush to get out before the park closed, I had skipped it.

And now that urge was nagging at me. I tried to ignore it, but it only grew stronger, until I was bursting with it. So even in the paradise that was Jemez Hot Springs, I was now feeling a pull to leave and head back to White Sands. Which is noteworthy, because it would take quite a bit for one to willfully cut short their stay in a place like Jemez.

This intuitive type of knowing, of feeling a pull, was born for me in Yolanthe's Kripalu yoga classes in Hoboken. Before Yolanthe invited me to hear and follow my intuition and my body's wisdom, I had made decisions only with my mind. I asked my mind if I was hungry or thirsty or attracted to someone. This led to such answers as, "I must be hungry, it's lunchtime," "Of course, I'm thirsty, it's 90 degrees out," and "I must be attracted to her, she looks like Gwyneth Paltrow."

But these are not necessarily *my* answers. They work sometimes, but not reliably. If it's lunchtime, I probably am hungry; if it's 90 degrees out, I probably do need a drink; and if she looks like Gwyneth, I probably am attracted to her. But not always. Kripalu invited me to ask not my mind but my body if I was hungry, thirsty, or attracted to someone. And surprisingly, it always gave me an answer. Before that I hadn't even realized that my body had a way of communicating. But it most certainly does. You can experience this too. Just sit in front of a pizza, a chocolate cake, a porn video, or someone else's poop, and your body will send you messages loud and clear.

Since then, I have felt a growing awareness of not only base urges but also of a subtler rightness or wrongness in all kinds of potential actions. When reaching for Brussels sprouts or even a tube of toothpaste in the grocery store, I often feel a pull, a neutrality, or an aversion.

Kripalu teaches practitioners to invite, hone, and follow these messages of pull, neutrality, or aversion. In new age circles we call this "following the energy," but that language can put some folks off and trigger references to Donald Sutherland in *Animal House* or Gary Busey in *Entourage*: "Can you *feel* the energy in the room, dude?"

If you try, though, you really can feel energies in a room. Next time you're in a tense fight with a partner or friend, take a moment to *feel* the quality of the space between the two of you in the room. And the next time things in your house or at work are joyous or productive, feel that space too. It's palpable.

Kripalu calls the energy that communicates pull, neutrality, and aversion *prana*. *Prana* is life force, *qi* in Chinese. It is an energy that "surrounds us and binds us. Luminous beings are we, not this crude matter. You must feel the Force around you; here, between you, me, the tree, the rock, everywhere.... Yes, even between the land and the ship."* Sorry. I think Yoda got it just right, though. And it worked for him — "When nine hundred years old *you* reach, look as good *you* will not, hmm?"

Prana craves the most intelligent path. It is what informs my sense of rightness or wrongness. When I reach for foods that heal and sustain me, *prana* pulls for them. When I contemplate a healthful

---

* From *Star Wars Episode V: The Empire Strikes Back*.

path that is in line with my values and allows for my growth, *prana* exerts an urge in that direction. *Prana* is as mysterious and yet, to me, as real as gravity itself.

On faith, simply because it felt right, I was beginning to give a lot of currency to urges and intuition. Kripalu teaches that the way to cultivate this is through experimentation and experience rather than through study — as they say, you can't transcend the mind by thinking; you can only go beyond the mind by stepping outside it. That is, the best way to cultivate and hone intuition is not by reading and planning and pondering, but by listening for and then following intuitions as they arise. As Malcolm Gladwell teaches in his bestseller *Blink*, each time you follow an intuition, your intuition strengthens.

So I had begun cultivating my sensitivity by inviting urges and then listening to them. And when I invited the messages, they would come. And if I ignored them, they'd get louder...and louder.

How can you tell if an urge is legitimate? First you follow the rules, the yogic Ten Commandments — the *yamas* and *niyamas*. If an urge violates a rule, you must ignore it — if you're angry and your urge is to hurt your brother, forget about it.

And second, for me, the litmus test for the legitimacy of an urge or intuition is to do yoga and meditate and see what happens. These practices quiet my mind and engage my heart and energy. If after yoga and meditation an urge or concern goes away, it was just a passing whim. But if during practice it builds and intensifies, and especially if all other thoughts fade away, leaving one urge shouting to be heeded, then I know I must follow it.

Such was the case here in Jemez. I soaked in the tubs. I practiced yoga and meditation. I communed with the trees. All that helped clear my mind, and eventually one and only one thought/feeling remained, and it was shouting, "White Sands!"

My mind disagreed with *prana* on this one, though, and thought that leaving Jemez was a terrible idea. It saw no reason to leave the luxurious hot springs and our new friends or to explain this cocka-mamie urge to Zach — Zach hated to backtrack, and we had just been at White Sands.

But I had to go, and I worked up the courage to speak to Zach.

"I have to return to White Sands," I told him.

"Drive three hundred miles back to White Sands? Why?"

"I have to do yoga there. I have a strong feeling about it."

"Uh-huh."

He was actually not that taken aback. He was used to this sort of *mishegas* by now, and anyway, he liked the plan as I pitched it to him: I would put him up at the youth hostel in Santa Fe, I'd be gone for one or two nights, and then I'd come back for him.

Zach and I left Jemez and headed to Santa Fe. The youth hos-tel was very cool, with a Southwestern-style open-air courtyard in the middle. Several twenty-something travelers were sitting on lawn chairs in the garden strumming guitars and taking breaks to eat jam on toast. One of the only downsides of sleeping in our van was that we rarely stayed in youth hostels.

It was odd to drive off alone as Zach waved good-bye, backpack and guitar case in hand, from the youth hostel driveway.

I hit the road and headed south for White Sands.

In my life now, with a family of four, I have to plan a five-hour road trip many weeks in advance, but back then, five hours seemed like a simple jaunt. At first. And then I knew I was on a spiritual quest, because twenty minutes later, as I cleared the back roads and entered the highway, Armageddon hit.

I drove right into a massive sandstorm. I thought these things existed only in *Roadrunner* cartoons, but my visibility was a few arm's lengths, and worse, I thought the van might actually tip.

In fact, it would not have taken much to tip that box of a van we drove. Recall that it was a 1990 Toyota Previa minivan. I am a huge fan of Toyota products, but 1990 was the first year Toyota produced a van. And it had a few kinks. For example, the oil was under the driver's seat. Literally. So checking the oil meant tipping the driver's seat back and finding the dipstick underneath.

And the van was about as sleek as my Great Aunt Birtha's permed coiffure. To challenge aerodynamics even further, Zach had absolutely insisted on bungee-cording two bulky, 1960s-era folded lawn chairs to the roof. Perhaps he imagined we'd attend an afternoon polka concert or a puppet show on a town common.

The chairs posed several problems. First of all, they gave the van a decidedly unfetching man-pushing-a-shopping-cart-with-all-his-possessions-in-it appearance, and I feared it wouldn't help us any with meeting women.*

Second, the bungee-corded lawn chairs hurt our gas mileage terribly. For ten thousand miles we just assumed the van handled and cornered like a shopping cart. In any kind of wind whatsoever, the driver needed two hands on the wheel, lest he lost control of the wild, bucking beast. But then after the first and only time we had need of the chairs, we accidentally left them behind, and we discovered that the van handled surprisingly well. It was not an Iroc-Z, mind you, but we could finally hit a corner at more than thirty miles an hour.

Unfortunately this epiphany happened weeks after my White Sands expedition, so as I navigated the sandstorm, my chair-sails

---

* To be fair, the chairs on top of this already very uncool box-like minivan also projected a family-on-their-way-to-Knott's-Berry-Farm vibe, which saved us from many police searches to which the beat-up, much cooler VW buses were continually subject. There's certainly no way we could have slept in so many four-star hotel parking lots in one of those. Basically, if you associate VW buses with dreadlocked Deadheads, then I'd say our van roughly correlated to your dad walking around the house in threadbare and possibly stained white boxer briefs, along with navy blue shin-high dress socks.

were aloft, and the beast was bucking like mad. I literally strained my biceps as I held the van on the road. The yellow median lines would have been meaningless to me, if I could have seen them. Thankfully, I was the only one on the road.

I finally made it to the White Sands National Monument and drove up to the visitor's gate. I must have looked a wreck. The ranger opened his booth window a crack and yelled through the wind, "I can let you in, but be careful. We'll have to close up if the sandstorm gets any worse."

Visibility was about thirty feet. I drove in and looked for the right place to pull over. I found a nice site for yoga. I fastened a bandanna over my mouth and nose to avoid breathing in sand and opened the door. Sand flooded into the van and stung the exposed skin on my face. I trudged out into the sand dune, though I stayed within site of the road and the van.

I started with a centering meditation and some chanting. I was pretty focused but noticed a ranger watching me. I think I was the only visitor during the storm, and he was watching me both for my own safety and so he could shut down the park and go home when I left. Perhaps, also, he was not used to someone doing yoga during a vicious sandstorm.

I did warm-ups and a few postures. Then I transitioned into a more intuitive practice, letting my body do what it wanted, following the flow of energy. This tapping into and following the flow of energy in the body is a hallmark of Kripalu yoga.

As I moved intuitively into and out of postures, flowing from one to the next, I found myself saying my name over and over again. This was an interesting practice; I so rarely say my own name. Try it right now. There is a strange power and awakening in saying your own name aloud.

I repeated my name over and over, and as I stood, I started to swing my arms like empty coat sleeves so they thumped against my body as they swung. I was acutely aware of my body and that it was me. I was aware of my breath and my sensations and my thinking. I felt more deeply embodied than ever before — usually I felt like a brain on a stick, and I welcomed moments of being present below the neck, but this was a new level of body consciousness.

Waking up my body would have been enough. But then I became aware of my environment — the sand, the sky, the wind — and I felt me in it too. And then came the huge leap, like the dissolving of a wall. I think it might have been the ominous, surreal, apocalyptic feeling of the white sandstorm that shook things up enough to bring about this insight and transcendence, because then I experienced all of it — the sand, the sky, the wind — as *me*.

I was not part of everything, but simply everything. I could feel the molecules of my consciousness inhabiting not just my body but everything around me as well.

The swinging of my arms became more rapid and more physical and the experience continued for a time, and then I started winding down and eventually came to a position lying on the ground. As I settled into relaxation pose, my consciousness and energy settled back into my body. I remembered being everything, but I was back in me.

After ten or so minutes of relaxation posture, I sat up to meditate. I felt the same way that I had after skydiving a year earlier, as if I had experienced a mental enema, my mind flushed clear. My meditation was not particularly deep or profound; I was just still and quiet and integrating.

Finally, I thanked the space for hosting me, had a moment of gratitude, and headed back to my van. Still integrating, I didn't feel like driving again in the storm. And I wondered if it was even safe in the dark (though the ranger assured me that nightfall would bring an ebbing of the winds).

I checked into a motel near the entrance to the park. I was a bit shaken, and I felt ungrounded and alone in the motel. I craved company and camaraderie.

In the morning everything was still, as if the previous day's cataclysm had never hit. I headed back to White Sands one more time to make sure my work there was done. I did not want to leave and then have to face Zach again with "I have to go back." But this time there was no pull. The park was once again just a national monument filled with a very interesting and somewhat mysterious gypsum sand dune. So I meditated, thanked the place again, and hit the road.

Five hours later I was in Santa Fe. I spent the day, until the designated meet-up time with Zach, looking around. Turns out he had spotted the van while I was strolling about and moved it to give me a scare. He definitely owed me that. The same storm that had turned White Sands into a maelstrom had given Santa Fe its latest springtime snowstorm in decades, and all Zach had were the clothes on his back, a change of underwear, and a light windbreaker.

Twenty-four hours earlier those light clothes were all Zach had seemed to need. But now, even though the snowstorm was over, it was 37 degrees and he was wearing every piece of clothing he had. So I suppose he was on the prowl in case he should spot the van and could get some warmer clothes out of it.

We met up at the ice-cream counter of the ancient Woolworth's in the center of town. We each had a story to tell. Then we headed west to Arizona.

∽

If I had ignored the pull that drew me back to White Sands, I never would have glimpsed oneness, and I surely would not have practiced yoga amid a raging desert sandstorm. Two items I can now happily check off my bucket list.

And, so, with that, ladies and gentlemen, let's say hello to our third Key to Happiness:

Cultivate and follow your intuition.

How do you do this? Start with Swami Kripalu and Malcolm Gladwell's advice: Listen for it, and then follow it.

That's how intuition grows.

This is not so different from following your bliss. In fact, I'd say following your bliss is a subset of following your intuition. Especially since intuition often communicates itself as a feeling of rightness. In the words of the late Steve Jobs, "Have the courage to follow your heart and intuition. They somehow already know what you truly want to become."*

I try to pose this question as often as possible, feel for an answer, and follow it. Every swami, yogi, researcher, and psychic that I've met gives this same piece of advice: The way to develop intuition is to listen for it and follow it.

Plus, relax and clear your mind. When you put mental chatter, ego, and personal desires aside and feel for what is really true, you see more clearly.

So friends, if you're playing along at home, here is your charge: Ask for and then follow your intuition as often as possible. Feel for what foods your body wants. Close your eyes and taste and sniff. Ask yourself on a day off from work, "What would feel just right today?" And at work, ask yourself, "What lights up my passion and makes me feel most alive?" Feel for a sense of rightness. You can even get full-on loony and walk around town asking *prana* to show you where to go. Feel for an unseen, energetic pull or aversion

---

* Commencement address, Stanford University, 2005.

drawing you in certain directions as you stroll. You might just have an unexpected adventure.

Oh, and by the way, you still have to follow the *yamas* and *niyamas*. They are your fail-safe that your "intuition" will not land you in front of a jury. Also, when you're unsure, get out your yoga mat or meditation cushion and get focused and quiet. See whether, with yoga and meditation, an urge or decision clarifies, builds, or goes away. Get in your body, engage your heart, invoke God or goodness, and see what happens. That should help you find and follow your intuition, and your bliss. Let us know your experiences at www.Misadventures-of-a-Yogi.com.

Chapter 15

Sedona, Arizona

The world is not only stranger than we imagine,
it is stranger than we can imagine.

— SIR ARTHUR STANLEY EDDINGTON, astronomer

I expected Sedona, Arizona, to be my Mecca. My macrobiotic aunt and a few yoga teachers had told me of Sedona's energy vortexes and its thriving new age community. I had been prepping Zach for weeks that I'd want to stay there for a while.

A vortex is a whirl, like a tornado or water going down a bathtub drain. The Sedona vortexes are believed to hold swirling energy that facilitates spiritual growth and transformation. The Sedona Chamber of Commerce describes the following kinds of vortexes: "Upflow Vortexes have energy flows that help you soar to higher spiritual perspectives...Inflow Vortexes have energy flows that help you go inward." As a full-fledged yogi/new ager I was pretty darned excited about all this. Even Zach, I think, was a bit curious.

Our first experience was outside Sedona at Slide Rock State Park. This place is a naturally occurring water park. People bathe in Oak Creek and slide down the slick red-rock rapids and waterfalls. It's Six Flags minus the chlorine. I frolicked for a while and then hiked away from the bustle to meditate and kick off our Sedona adventure.

We drove into Sedona at lunchtime and selected a Chinese buffet in a strip mall. Heralding our stay in Sedona, I found a large bug in my food. I was repulsed, but Zach was overjoyed because the management comped both our meals. If he'd had tweezers and a Baggie, I'm sure Zach would have harvested the bug to use in restaurants across the country. We'd have been national scofflaws, the Bonnie and Clyde of free lunches.

Next we pulled into a motel bearing the sign Hiring Maids. We figured that we'd stay in Sedona for at least a week and that maybe we would make some traveling money. We were willing to work for very little. We met with the manager, but he decided that by the time he trained us we'd be leaving, so it was not worth his while. It was a bit of an ego blow, but I understood his reasoning.

By now, after a few hours in Sedona, Zach and I both acknowledged that we were "feeling something." We felt "weird." Might have been the MSG in our Chinese food. Might have been the placebo of expectations. Might have been the clear, dry desert air or even just the look of the Mars-like red rocks surrounding Sedona.

What happened next is a blur and culminated with us hiking a mountain with six strangers to sit around a fire and chant through the night. Here's what I remember.

I looked in my yoga directory to find a class and selected one that appealed. The address led us to a small house at the foot of a scrubby desert mountain at the edge of town. We knocked on the door, and when a woman opened it, we asked for the yoga class. She told us to come back on Tuesday at 4:00 pm. We told us about our trip. She had us in for tea and suggested a hike beginning at a trailhead down the street.

We took the hike through scrubby desert paths and were deposited in front of a crystal shop on a main road a mile or so from her house. We went into the shop and browsed. We were accosted by a giant of a woman who ran the shop. If we had been on the set of Will

Smith's *Men in Black*, she'd certainly have been one of the aliens. Actually, she looked an awful lot like Hagrid's girlfriend Madame Olympe Maxime, headmistress of Beauxbatons Academy of Magic. And she was overflowing with advice and predictions. She told us we *needed* to speak with a man named Eberly at Eberly's Crystal Emporium.

We walked back to the van and drove to the other crystal shop. We found Eberly, and next thing I know, we're hiking Sedona's famous Bell Rock, one of the most renowned vortex sites, with six strangers, all of us toting *djembe* drums and jugs of water.

The drumming and chanting were nice. Not radically transformational, but nice. Actually it was less nice for Zach. Recall that Zach is an accomplished a cappella singer and musician. This was his first experience with spiritual chanting, and he had no problem with that vibe, but he kept searching for harmony. And there ain't no harmony among a bunch of nonmusicians chanting and banging on *djembes*. To me it all sounded rich and transcendent, but to a musically trained ear, these dissonant, cacophonous "ahhoohhhhmmmms" can get under the skin. He kept trying to provide the perfectly pitched "om" to unite the noise of the group into one. I'd open my eyes every now and then to find Zach contorting his mouth, looking frantically around the circle, and pointing at different members of the group, as though conducting a zombie chorus or attempting hopelessly to juggle seven balls. By the end, he was frazzled and exhausted.

I showed Zach this chapter and he told me that I left part of the story out. Apparently, that evening, after the chanting, things got pretty weird. Eberly gave a long and trippy lecture about aliens, UFOs, and abductions. I remember none of this. Come to think of it, I can't account for about five hours of my time that night.

Besides this unnerving fact, the most exceptional thing I can say about my experience in Sedona is how rapidly we moved from one lead to another. In most towns we might or might not meet a local. But we had never been cast from one happenstance to another so rapidly, like characters in a mystery film, like Robert Langdon and Sophie Neveu in *The Da Vinci Code*. It was quite a whirlwind experience.

The next day we wandered around Sedona with less effect. We spent the night in the van at the summit of Bell Rock, and in the morning we hit the road. We had definitely felt something in Sedona. No huge epiphanies, but something.

We had been in Sedona for only thirty-six hours, and we were ready to move on. I had planned for Sedona to be the apex of my trip. Another reminder to be present to what actually unfolds. I think I shall again quote Amrit Desai, who said, "The more beliefs and conclusions you have about life, the less you are willing to explore the infinite wealth and beauty of [what actually happens]."

You can't know or plan for where you'll find transcendence; you can only follow the whispers as they call out to you.

Chapter 16

Belting Out the Bhagavad Gita

The greatest thing you'll ever learn
is just to love and be loved in return.

— EWAN MCGREGOR, *Moulin Rouge!*, 2001

*B*esides Sedona, all I remember about our time in Arizona are some very, very good corn tortillas. We bought a pig pack of a hundred and ate them for a week. The tortillas were homemade, and whether we ate them with salsa or peanut butter, those things were sublime. Zach's favorite was peanut butter, raisins, bananas, and some of the honey that John and Annie had given us in Hot Springs all rolled up into a delicious little taco.

After Arizona we crossed into southern California and headed straight for San Diego. I checked my yoga directory, and right outside San Diego, in La Jolla Beach, I found Svaroopa yoga at Master Yoga Academy. This style is now pretty popular around the country, but it was all started right there by Rama Berch, now known as Swami Nirmalananda Saraswati, on Fay Avenue in La Jolla.

The Svaroopa class was sumptuous. It was not as overtly free-spirited as Yolanthe's Kripalu classes — no one farted or moaned or spoke in tongues during postures, and we didn't begin the class by sharing about our day — but it was sweet. It was slow and gentle and deep and compassionate and the instructor was cute and my muscles melted.

I bought a class card and attended every day. I was relaxed and my body felt great, and I thought, "Maybe this is my new yoga style; maybe I'll do their teacher training," but my heart, while contented, did not sing at the possibility.

By the time we arrived in San Diego, Zach was running out of traveling money. He had anticipated this and had a plan. At home in New Jersey, he had registered with a few national temp agencies so that he could temp for a week or two in California. He contacted the agency and secured a week's placement in San Diego.

Zach donned his one tie and traded his guitar case in for a make-shift briefcase (his backpack), while I headed north to Grass Valley, California, for a week's work exchange at an ashram. I would work in barter for room, board, and yoga.

Zach surveyed his new office building and discovered that California, always an environmental step ahead of the rest of the country, encourages businesses to have a shower on premises so that employees can bike to work. Zach's plan was to sleep in the van in the parking lot, shower in the building, put on the one white shirt, and tie, that he had packed, and go to work. He spent his evenings on the beach or at the local reciprocal gym.

Zach's coworkers must have gotten a kick out of their new one-tie-wearing friend. I imagine that behind his back they either mocked him or spoke of him in reverent tones. Perhaps he is a legend still in the mythos of the place, the guy who lived in the parking lot for a week. And I bet his employer got more than they planned for in that week. Zach is ultra-talented and super-hardworking (he is now an executive at a major corporation), so I'm sure he surprised more than a few people with his output.

Zach made $300. That may not be much to a family with

children, but to Zach, living out of the van and eating peanut butter sandwiches, it bought another month on the road.

While Zach worked for the man, I was volunteering at a Sivananda yoga ashram. Throughout the trip I had found classes in all kinds of yoga styles, from gentle restorative to power Vinyasa ashtanga. I had practiced in churches, libraries, college gyms, parks, and cafés. And now I was excited to spend some time in an ashram.

The only ashram I had been to up till then was Kripalu. The Kripalu Center for Yoga and Health in Lenox, Massachusetts, is very large. On a busy weekend it houses more than six hundred guests. So I was surprised when I called the Grass Valley Sivananda Yoga Farm and the head of the ashram answered the phone. I was even more surprised when he offered to pick me up at the bus station.

Misha showed up and was no disappointment. He had wild gray-blond hair and unkempt, food-stained clothes; he was a bit overweight; and he chanted Sanskrit to himself constantly. And man, this guy was deep; the real deal. As soon as Misha picked me up, I became part of his small ashram family. Most people in a place that receives new weekly volunteers protect themselves from the inevitable loss of transient friends by generally ignoring volunteers and sticking exclusively with the long-term residents. But Misha was present. When I was there, I was his brother. He simply enjoyed being human and connecting with other humans. He was like my five-year-old son enjoying a new friend made at a playground, unconcerned about, or even aware of, tomorrow.

Misha chanted, asked me questions, and laughed quite a bit as we drove. Then we were home, and he pulled into the long ashram driveway. I was stunned by the quiet beauty of the place. The ashram consisted of a farmhouse and several outbuildings nestled into a picturesque valley of softly rolling hills, covered by pastel-green grass.

Misha parked his van near the ashram's extremely generous compost heap. This beast was overflowing with brown rice, beans, greens, orange rinds, and banana slugs. I had never seen a real banana slug before. These giant gastropods toe a perfect line between cough-up-your-lunch-vile and so-cute-I-want-to-pet-one. They are entirely too large to exist in New Jersey, where we require all our bugs to measure in at no more than one inch, crown to rump. There's paperwork and weekly check-ins, like with prostitutes in Amsterdam. So these six-inch-long critters would never cut it. They'd be hunted by a midnight posse and eliminated.

As soon as we pulled into the ashram, Misha was called away on official business, and since I was transfixed watching the compost heap, I was left alone to find my way. I walked to the main house. While Misha was my new brother, I was not his new favorite. As soon as I was out of his sight, he was present with his next task or interaction.

And not everyone welcomed me with the open heart of Misha. In fact, once I got into the house, no one welcomed me at all. This was not a spa-shram, as we devoted Kripaluites jokingly refer to Kripalu, so there was no front desk, no inviting samovar of tea or silver bowl of fruit to welcome me, no information binders, and no protocol for checking in new volunteers.

I wandered around. Misha was likely now outside shoveling compost while humming a tune from the Gita, and everyone else probably assumed I had already been shown around. So I was alone. I had been on the road for six weeks, and I was feeling lost. I missed my family and I missed things familiar. I missed knowing my way around. I was tired of everything being new. I also felt free, as if I was experiencing a deeper me, one that was beneath the usual routines and habits. But in that moment I felt very alone.

Finally, Misha's number two, Priti, found me. We had lunch, and then Misha assigned everyone's postlunch chores. He asked me to mow the lawn, but I had no closed-toed shoes (which was really just an excuse to avoid admitting that I had never actually used a lawn mower and was afraid of it — I am Jewish and from northern New Jersey, and I think you'll be hard-pressed to find a Jew born and raised in northern New Jersey who knows how even to pull the cord on a gas mower; we find them very intimidating).

Instead, I got the job of cleaning the toilets. Obviously, I was also terrified of these bacteria dragons, and I stretched my arms as long as possible to avoid being spritzed in the face as I cleaned. But at least these were environmentally friendly composting toilets, and the cleanser was organic, fresh-smelling Dr. Bronner's peppermint castile soap.

After work we had dinner. A friend of the ashram, James, aka Satyananda to his yoga friends, showed up with fresh chard from his garden. Everyone was very excited, but I had no idea what chard was. In 1995, unless you lived on a commune or in California, you had never eaten a green other than spinach, iceberg lettuce, and maybe the very mysterious escarole in Progresso Escarole Soup.

Satyananda and that day's designated cook put together a great meal, and we ate outside. Misha ate by himself, eyes closed, lost in blissful reverie, and Priti was involved with ashram business, so I ate alone.

That night I was shown my room. No joke, this "room," in the attic of the house, had a ceiling four feet high and was slightly larger than the antique twin mattress it housed. My one roommate was a mushroom growing right out of the floorboards. That night I wept. I wept because I was so alone. I wept because I was three hundred miles from Zach, the only person on this coast who knew me. I wept because I was a mold- and bacteriaphobe sleeping next to a giant fungus. (I was afraid that if I took my eyes off this thing for even a moment, it would walk toward me.) I cried myself to sleep.

When I woke up I was cleaned out. I was also, it turns out, in some trouble. Life at a Sivananda yoga center follows a strict flow. Up at 5:30. Chant and meditate till 8:00. Yoga at 8:00. Breakfast, chores, lunch, chores, yoga, dinner, evening chanting, bedtime. In my attic cell, I had slept through the morning wake-up call, and I stumbled into the main room during meditation. Misha chided me.

Misha assigned the day's work, and I was assigned cleaning out the second story of an old building. It was infested with cat poop, and I think this particular chore may have been a punishment for oversleeping. I didn't mind too much, though, because I was paired for the job with a new volunteer, Frederique, a young French woman who had arrived that morning, a week early for a monthlong yoga teacher training program.

To this garden state yogi, Frederique was very mysterious and very sexy. She spoke with a French accent, she was empowered, referring to herself as a woman, not a girl, and she was tall and a bit beefy. I imagined that back home she drank a lot of fresh whole milk and wandered the hills in overalls and pig tails herding sheep and gathering wildflowers.

Frederique and I swept dust and copious cat poop. This was easily, hands down, one of the vilest jobs of my life, probably not even safe without full hazmat paraphernalia, but Frederique's cuteness trumped my bacteriaphobia, and she and I joked around as we moved about in the clouds of dust and desiccated cat poop and had a great old time. It was like *Little House* when Pa assigned Half Pint and Manly to clean out the barn, with the two young'uns laughing, having a hay fight, and smearing cow shit on each other's work clothes.

To my surprise, not much actual practice of yoga postures went on that week at the ashram. We chanted, we meditated, we ate organic local food, we mindfully performed manual labor as *seva* (selfless service). We lived a beautiful, simple life in as beautiful and serene a setting as I've ever seen, but we never so much as touched our toes, let alone plumbed the depths of *paschimottanasana* (seated forward bend). During the 4:00 PM scheduled yoga time everyone lazed on the lawn, had a dip in the lake, soaked in some sun on the dock, or went off to do their own thing.

Actually, one resident did do yoga every day at the designated time. His name was Hansel, and he lived by himself on the hillside in a tiny hut that he had built by hand — he was a former architect who had retired in midlife to the ashram.

Hansel's hut was not much bigger than my attic cubby. And Hansel was uncharacteristically surly for an ashram denizen. I think there was somehow some bad blood between Misha and him. Misha was completely civil and probably faultless in the discord, but anything he said to Hansel was met with the sort of angsty reply you expect only from a teenager to his or her parents. If a mom said to her sixteen-year-old, "Have fun at the party, honey. Can I walk you in?" the teen's reply would sound exactly like everything Hansel said to Misha. Hansel was the constant heckler to Misha's show. And since he was no more cordial to me, the new guy, I did not join him for his daily yoga practice. I was therefore disappointed to do yoga entirely on my own at the ashram.

One of the highlights of my week at the ashram was our trip to the movies. I'd always romanticized what it must have been like to live in the communes of the sixties and seventies, on Ram Dass's farm or at Swami Satchidananda's ashram. And after months on the road, I wanted a home, a group of friends to be part of. I wanted Ken Kesey, though I'd have settled for Jerry, George, Kramer, and Elaine. And our ashram field trip to the movies dropped me right into a yogic version of the Merry Pranksters' school bus.

We all piled into the ashram van and made for the town cinema. We were headed to see *Dorothy Parker and the Vicious Circle*, an indie film, because Misha didn't like the violence and sexuality of mainstream Hollywood movies. I can see that these would be too intense or perhaps too sexually stimulating for him, a celibate renunciate. And no tapes, radio, or CDs for us on the way there, either. Misha led us in devotional Sanskrit *bhajans*. We chanted the Bhagavad Gita like Wayne and Garth belting out "Bohemian Rhapsody." Sitting next to Frederique in the back of that van, I could not have been happier.

A few days later, my weeklong stay was over, and Misha was driving me back to the bus station. We knew each other pretty well by then.

"You are a *sadhak* — a seeker," he said, "a true yogi, and you should stay with us. Why are you leaving?"

"Because you don't do yoga," I replied.

My response was honest and without barb or resentment, and Misha just nodded. But now, years later, I see that Misha did yoga every moment of every day without ever unrolling a sticky mat. He was present as he ate, present as he worked, and present as he played. He was ever committed to God, chanting her name throughout the day. And most important, he faced every interaction and every moment with a full and open heart.

Chapter 17

San Francisco

God has prepared a path for everyone to follow.
You just have to read the omens that he left you.

— PAULO COELHO, *The Alchemist*

I arrived in San Francisco three days before Zach was scheduled
to arrive. We had a voice mail back home in New Jersey where
we could leave each other messages — this was before cell phones
— and I understood that he had finished pimping for the man and
was making his way in the van up the 550 miles of Highway 1 from
San Diego to San Francisco. It was on that stretch of road where
Zach had his epiphany.

The beautiful scenery moved him. Highway 1 is like no other
highway — with its mountain-hugging byways overlooking the
ocean, lavender and crimson sunsets, and the circus sights of Ven-
ice Beach — and during the drive, the shining beauty of the place
burned through the fog of his malaise and woke him up.

Zach realized that while he enjoyed these sights alone, he longed
to share them with someone. Zach opened up. He was done mourning his heartbreaks and professional disappointments. He was ready
to find someone to share his life with. He was ready to invest himself
in a career. At this point, for Zach, the trip was complete. He had
found what he was looking for, and the rest was just for fun.

When we got home, Zach found an apartment in New York City and set up a life, one warmly entwined with the lives of others. It was not long before he began a successful career, and not long before he met his soul mate, Rachel. They are now married with two children.

Until Zach arrived in San Francisco, I stayed at the Union Square Youth Hostel. I had a great routine. I ate breakfast at the hostel or in the small diner downstairs, I read Paulo Coelho's *The Alchemist* in cafés or in Golden Gate Park, and I explored the city and its many yoga offerings. I took classes at the Integral Yoga Institute in the Mission District and at the Sivananda Yoga Vedanta Center on Arguello Boulevard, right next to Golden Gate Park, and I found a studio that was not dedicated to one style but offered everything from Shamanic yoga to tai chi–inspired Chi yoga.

In San Francisco it's no surprise that "fearless, honest, relaxed" brought me many adventures. For example, in my previous life as a sedate private school math teacher in New Jersey, I certainly would not have gotten into the Cadillac of a man I had met naked in a yoga center locker room, even if he offered to bring me to his chiropractic office for a free session. And this would certainly be especially true if his name were Dr. Sweetmember. But two repetitions of "fearless, honest, relaxed," and there I was in Dr. Sweetmember's Caddie headed to Fort Mason.

Was I nervous? Yes. But my intuition told me that it was okay. And my intuition was tested several times in San Francisco. Another time when I was traveling in the city's splendid underground/overground metro system, a churlish homeless chap in a wheelchair asked me to push him to the elevator. I was proud of myself for being of service. I was Russell, Wilderness Explorer extraordinaire, helping Ed Asner's *UP* curmudgeon, and thrilled for the opportunity to do a good deed and get my merit badge.

We followed signs around several increasingly dark corners and reached the elevator, where we were noticeably and, I must shamefully admit, uncomfortably very alone. My spidey senses were tingling, and I wanted out of there as soon as possible. He asked me to push him in. I did. He then asked me to ride with him, to get into the elevator and accompany him up to the next floor. My spidey senses shouted, "No!" I'm not sure if this was actual intuition of danger or bourgeois bigotry, but I could not get into that elevator. Plus, it made no good sense, really. He could reach the elevator buttons. He could get out on his own, and then he'd be at the surface with lots of people around to help him if needed. I did not need to be alone with him for the ride.

I also realized that I might have looked the perfect target: idealistic, wide-eyed, map-wielding young traveler looking confused and in no rush. I said no, and he cursed profusely at me as I walked back to the subway platform.

But when Dr. Sweetmember, naked in the locker room, asked me after a particularly moving yoga class if he could give me a free chiropractic session, I saw no red flags. I got in his Caddie, and we drove from the Mindful Body yoga center to his office. He told me about the city as we drove. Deep down I felt safe, but still my mind ran scenarios of me rolling to a stop after jumping, Bond-like, from the moving car.

When we got to his office and I saw the framed photos of the good doctor with famous LA Lakers such as Magic Johnson and Kareem Abdul-Jabbar, I knew I was okay. He set me up on a pre-adjustment chiropractic table, pressed a button, and went to make a few phone calls.

I don't know if all chiropractors' tables are like this, but his table jimmied and jerked in an attempt to relax my muscles, or perhaps just to catch them off guard. I lay on the contraption for what seemed like fifteen minutes until I was thoroughly shaken and stirred. Then he came in and gave me an adjustment, followed by a taste of royal jelly, a special honey reserved for the queen bee that is sold to a cult-like following in health food stores. Guy at the Hoboken Harvest would have been very pleased.

Dr. Sweetmember finished the session and seemed to be delaying my departure. There did not seem to be any ulterior motive other than wanting to hang out longer with me. He asked if I'd come back for a free follow-up.

As I prepared to leave, I asked him, Why all the free treatment? Why did he invite me in the locker room? Why me, a total stranger?

Even with Magic and Kareem watching over us, his answer freaked me out a bit.

"You are a Jewish fellow, yes?" he asked.

"Um, yes."

"Our savior was Jewish, and you look like him," was all the reason he needed.

Indeed, I was sporting a giant beard, longish hair, a thin frame and face, an olive tan, and certainly a wide-eyed and open look. Plus, I was still riding the high of my White Sands unity experience and Jerry's green light. I was only missing Oskar's flowing white robes.

In a different situation Dr. Sweetmember's rationale might have sent me running for the street, but in the office of this kindly, if a bit batty, chiropractor it was perfect. I also knew I had another great story for Zach, and one that this time, thankfully, involved no offer of "special services."

❧

For me, like Zach, the trip essentially ended in San Francisco. Or more specifically, it ended on California Street at the Mindful Body, the same yoga studio where I met Dr. Sweetmember. Because after taking classes in Power yoga, Iyengar yoga, Sivananda yoga, Shamanic yoga, Chi yoga, and Integral yoga, I eventually showed up for a Kripalu yoga class.

The teacher was new to this center, so she didn't have much of a following yet, and only one other guy showed up. She almost canceled the class but ran it at our behest.

I expected little from her, since she was a brand-new teacher. We started with an "om" and headed into warm-ups. Right away, the familiar opening, language, and warm-ups transported me into the attic of the Hoboken Harvest. I could almost see and hear Yolanthe in the room, could smell Guy's Sunshine Burgers on the grill. My body and mind responded, and I was at ease and at home in a way I had not been for the past two months on the road. And furthermore, Dina, the teacher, was right-on. She had recently completed Kripalu yoga teacher training and was attentive and insightful and so very present with her heart as she taught.

She included all the Kripalu trademarks. We did the Breath of Joy warm-up. Dina invited us to tune in and listen to our body's wisdom and guidance. We held a simple posture for an extended time and watched the sensation and energy build in our bodies as we breathed into any discomfort. And then we released the posture and allowed our bodies to flow intuitively through stretches or postures. Dina even played soothing music of bamboo flutes and birds chirping.

Even before we did the pigeon posture (my favorite yoga posture, which I had experienced, so far, only in Kripalu classes), I knew. I knew that whatever Amrit's transgressions had been, this style of yoga spoke to me. It relaxed my body and opened my heart. In a Kripalu yoga class I felt held and supported.

After Dina's class, I called the Kripalu toll-free number and enrolled myself in their next monthlong residential teacher training.

Years later I bumped into Dina at Kripalu. She still lived in San

Francisco and was in the Berkshires taking a continuing ed training at the mother ship. I had been to her class only that one time, five years earlier, but since it had been one of her first, she remembered me. We chatted for a few minutes, and I was happy finally to share with her that her class had brought me back to Kripalu yoga.

Chapter 18

Ayurveda Revisited

> When diet is wrong, medicine is of no use.
> When diet is correct, medicine is of no need.
>
> — Ayurvedic proverb

After San Francisco we headed home, which was three thousand miles away. We passed through Nevada, the only state where Ruby could practice her craft legally, through Utah, where we were kicked out of Dinosaur National Monument by a very friendly ranger for sleeping in a parking lot, through Colorado, the most beautiful state, I'd say, apart from California, which isn't even fair to count, and through Nebraska, which, I'm sorry to report, smelled exactly like cow shit for the entire length of the state. In fact, if you want to be convinced to eat only grass-fed, humanely raised beef, try driving through Nebraska during slaughter season and drive past the pens of cattle standing hoof deep in their own feces.

I can't remember Iowa very well; perhaps I slept through it while Zach drove. And then, one day, we were in Chicago.

In Chicago, we stayed with a friend of Zach's who was in a master's program at the University of Chicago. We wandered through the Art Institute, and we ate excellent deep-dish pizza at Giordano's.

And in a bookstore near the university, I found the Ayurvedic cookbook that I mentioned back in Hot Springs, Arkansas.

Zach and his buddy sat for hours and reminisced. This friend of Zach's is, by the way, of note because his first name rhymes with his last name, putting him at great advantage if he decides to become a notable musician, porn star, or serial killer.

So while Zach and Rick Dick (see what I mean) caught up, I spent many hours in cafés reading and taking notes from my new book. The book began with a forty-six-page introduction about Ayurveda. I learned that according to Ayurveda an individual is a blend of three proclivities, or *doshas*, described as ether/air (*vata*), fire (*pitta*), and water/earth (*kapha*). Each person is characterized by a unique blend of these energies. Ayurveda posits that health and vitality result from respecting the particular needs and maximizing the innate gifts of one's *dosha*. Translation: if spicy food aggravates you, don't eat it, and if beans give you horrendous gas, eat them a bit less often.

I learned that a person with lots of ether/air (me) is often very creative and funny and flexible (if I do say so myself), but when out of balance can become overly creative, overly flexible, and overly airy — basically, scatterbrained, wishy-washy, and flatulent (d'oh!).

The book gave a tongue-in-cheek introduction stating, essentially, that if you want to keep *vata* unbalanced, then worry, don't get enough sleep, eat on the run, keep no routine, eat dry or leftover foods, drive around a lot, and repress your feelings. D'oh, again! On the road, I was seven for seven.

I decided to take immediate evasive action and begin a regime of *vata* balancing. The book told me that in order to keep *vata* balanced, I needed to keep warm, eat warm and moist foods, take it easy on beans, avoid white sugar and processed foods, relax, spend lots of time in nature, and keep a regular routine.

Interestingly, one of the two coauthors of the book was Urmila Desai, Amrit's wife. And Amrit (Kripalu's former guru) had written the foreword. Looked like he was still to be in my life after all.

୰

And here we come to our fourth Key to Happiness:

Apply at least three pieces of Ayurvedic wisdom to your daily schedule.

You won't regret it. Begin by turning to appendix 6 to determine your Ayurvedic constitution. Then, in appendix 7, choose at least three recommendations for your type. (Yes, this may involve massaging sesame oil at every orifice of your body, and no, you will not be required to use sesame oil enemas.) Let us know how it goes at www.Misadventures-of-a-Yogi.com.

BOOK THREE

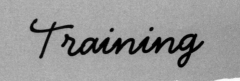

Training

Chapter 19

Cotton Swabs

Health depends on being in harmony with our souls.
— DR. EDWARD BACH

*W*hen Zach dropped me off at my parents' house, I said good-bye to him and imagined it was for good. Seventy days together, and I was done. But by the next day when he called to invite me to help out at his mom's garage sale, I was eager to get together. I loved this guy like a brother. He knew me better at that point than anyone else, and after twelve thousand miles on the road, he had heard all my stories and knew all my secrets.

Our quirky Toyota Previa minivan also had heard all my stories and knew all my secrets. The van had served us well, had been our home for more than two months. But we were done with it, and since we both needed some cash, Zach sold the van at his mom's garage sale. Zach is a truly brilliant salesman. I mean, who sells a van at a garage sale? Old Dungeons & Dragons Monster Manuals, yes. Polynesian-themed salt and pepper shakers, surely. But a van?

Zach had spent the whole morning prepping the van and removing twelve thousand miles of grime. He disassembled the futon and put the seats back in. He personally detailed every surface, even using Q-tips to dust inside the dashboard's air-conditioning and heating vents.

Q-tips, by the way, epitomize the very delusion that I am fighting in this world. It's not that I hate Q-tips; I love them, that cleaned-out, the-world-is-good feeling I get when I swab my ears after a shower. But I resent that every box housing cotton swabs advises against using them in your ears. Everyone knows that's what you use them for. It's why you buy them. And the cotton swab companies know this. Everyone in America, besides my wife, who is from Canada and actually adheres to rules and regulations on boxes, ignores this.*

After the warning on the cotton swabs box, there are helpful hints about what these fitting-in-your-ear-perfectly devices are actually for: applying ointment, baby care, household cleaning, and cleaning computer keyboards. When's the last time you actually used them to dust between the keys on your laptop (especially ever since Aunt Edna gave you that very thoughtful novelty keyboard vac from Brookstone)?

So what I disapprove of is the lie we are all living. I seek to erase the lie, to live in truth and honesty, to remove the dissonance between reality and what I tell myself.

By the way, it's not that the box is wrong. An ear, nose, and throat doctor friend of mine hates cotton swabs. He once told me that they are responsible for half the ear problems he sees: cotton swabs can cause micro cuts in the wall of the ear canal, which can later get infected; they can push wax to build up in the ear (left to its own devices the ear will actually rid itself of excess wax); and

---

* Yes, Canadians are obscenely rule abiding and polite. Here's an example. At a fancy restaurant my wife won't use the cloth restaurant napkin to blow her nose. Can you believe it? She will only use a tissue or paper napkin. Unbelievable! What's that? Really? You won't use a restaurant's cloth napkin either? Oh, great, now I look like a cretin.

sometimes the cotton tip falls off and the doctor has to fish it out with forceps.

So since cotton swabs are apparently the bane of ear health, the warning is totally warranted, and I don't have a problem with that at all. I have a problem with the lie we all complicitly live with. I have a problem with cotton swab *don't ask, don't tell*. It is an insult to authenticity. This is a severe *yama* and *niyama* violation, people. How pranically draining is it to use cotton swabs with that warning staring right at you?

On that day in May, however, Zach used his Q-tips by the book. He was probably the one person that year in our town to use them properly.

And somehow he sold the van to a family for $4,500. We had purchased it for $5,000. After traveling to California and back, we were short only $500 (and a whole lot of gas money, more than needed because of those motherfunchin' lawn chairs).

I planned to stay at my parents' house for the two months until yoga teacher training began in July. And three days into my stay, my folks left for a two-week vacation, so I was able to manifest my commune fantasy, as college friends from around the globe flew in and lived at my house. At any given moment there were veggie dogs on the grill, Wiffle ball on the lawn, yoga in the den, and a game of basketball in the pool. Friends slept on every bed, sofa, and carpeted floor in the house. One woman, late to arrive and claim her spot, made a nest of towels and sheets she had found in the linen closet.

During my two months at Mom and Dad's, I prepared for yoga teacher training. Bikram yoga, a very challenging form of yoga practiced in a super-heated room, had become increasingly popular at Kripalu, and I was worried that it had infiltrated my otherwise gentle style of yoga. I wondered if Bikram's voice, "Puuuuush! Good. Now push further!" had seeped ever so subtly into Kripalu's afternoon yoga practice. I wanted to make sure I was up to the task, so I bought a cassette tape of a formal Bikram class and practiced with the tape one afternoon...and passed out. Truly. Thus, my pre-Kripalu training regimen.

For those two months, I trained. I played chess with neighborhood friends. And I spent time with my younger sister, Julie — she and I were making a transition from siblings to inseparable friends. Together, we were simultaneously discovering our interests in hiking, yoga, meditation, and holistic health. We toured every health food market, holistic shop, crystal emporium, metaphysical bookstore, and yoga center in Bergen County, New Jersey. This was not as difficult as it sounds, though, since in 1995 there were only seven such places in the county. We had a great time of it. We'd explore new paths in the woods of the Ramapo Reservation, we'd try out yoga classes, and we'd sit together in a café thoroughly chewing our brown rice.

After two blissful months of carefree Mom-and-Dad's-house living, I packed up my sweats and headed to Kripalu. I drove the scenic Taconic Parkway north through bucolic countryside and past diners with mirrored cases offering fourteen kinds of pie. I had my usual Beavis and Butthead–style laugh as I passed through Coxsackie, New York, and after two and a half hours, I arrived at Kripalu.

I checked in, was assigned my room, and selected my bunk. Actually, I wasn't really *assigned* a room, per say, since all men slept in the same room. Back then, Kripalu, like yoga in general, attracted mostly women. So most of the dorms throughout the giant four-story building were used to house women, and all the men were lumped together in a large one-room ghetto. The women slept in small, genteel suites, while the men slept forty-eight to a room. For privacy, some men hung blankets or sheets over clotheslines suspended between bunks, so the room had a shantytown quality to it. I selected a bottom bunk near a window and was very happy to be there.

Our schedule was morning yoga at 5:30 AM, breakfast, morning program, lunch, afternoon program, dinner, evening program or free time, and sleep. We would do that for thirty days in a row. It was marvelous.

As it turned out, I was more than prepared for the Bikram-polluted afternoon yoga classes and would have been even without the extra training. The taint was ever so slight, and the class remained the gentle Kripalu style that I craved. Bikram's voice saying, "Puuuuush! Good. Now push furtherrrr!" had been filtered through Kripalu-speak and turned into, "Now close your eyes, bring your consciousness into your hip, and explore the joint with tiny micromovements." It was the difference between a New Yorker pulling out a tire iron when you've accidentally stolen his parking spot and an Englishman saying, "Excuse me, I believe I arrived first, now there's a good chap."

There really is, by the way, something called Kripalu-speak. It's a gentle way of speaking and a certain, unmistakable teaching language, called *languaging* in yoga teacher circles. Whereas a teacher in an Iyengar class might say, "No, that's wrong. Rotate your right hip three degrees inward and pull up through your psoas," Kripalu people would say, "Close your eyes, bring your consciousness into your right hip, and explore the joint with tiny micromovements."

And in Kripalu-speak, the ubiquitous saffron-and-pink cushions at Kripalu that are used in meditation and as bolsters during yoga postures are called *Kri-pillows*. And Kripalu people — the folks you see walking the halls on any given visit, much like the extras on *Fantasy Island* or *The Love Boat* — are called *Kri-people*.

My monthlong yoga teacher training spanned July to August, when, in the Berkshires, it gets pretty hot. There was no air-conditioning in the classrooms, which I actually didn't mind at all — I wouldn't want to do breathing exercises or yoga postures in air-conditioned air, anyway. But when I showed up to afternoon yoga class wearing my sweats, I was *shvitzing*. So the next morning I wore a pair of Umbro soccer shorts and boxers — at the time I wore boxers exclusively; they seemed much more chill than the tightie-whities of my adolescence.

But I had never done yoga in Umbro shorts and boxers in a class before, so I didn't see it coming as I bared my soul and my manhood to the class in shoulder stand posture that day. So on our first break I headed to town to get something more discreet.

Kripalu is nestled in the town of Lenox, Massachusetts, which also houses Tanglewood, the summer home of the Boston Pops. As a result, Lenox is filled with very upscale boutiques airlifted straight from SoHo or Fifth Avenue, and the only undies I found were Calvin Kleins for $40 a three-pack. So for the next yoga class I was tucked safely into my Calvins.

My month at Kripalu kept me more removed from pop culture than I had ever been. Apart from my trip to Lenox for undies and a sojourn to Friendly's that included two classmates and I "om"-ing in unison to bless our meal, I never left the grounds. I watched no TV. I saw no billboards or movie previews. And I never saw a *Glamour* or *People* magazine. Whereas when I first arrived I was comparing everyone to Brad Pitt and Gwyneth Paltrow (engaged to each other at the time), by the end I saw people as they were. Not because I had changed so much, I think, but because I was not filled with so many pop-culture images. This was an amazing experience, because I found that people as they are, whether with blotchy skin, wrinkled skin, red hair, silver hair, no hair, flat bellies, fat bellies, smooth feet, or stinky feet are actually very interesting and unique and beautiful.

The Kripalu Center was in transition back then. It was still an ashram even without its excommunicated guru, but it was finding and redefining itself. People were hurt and confused, and most of the devotional practices, such as chanting, had been dropped —

the Kri-people were angry and weren't sure who to chant to. Some wanted to toughen up, so martial arts became very popular for a time.

Even with the changes, the old rules were technically still in place. Every dorm room and most coffee tables, end tables, and information stations still had the "binder of rules," an exhaustive tome of do's and don'ts.

I had read the binder with the earnest intention of following the rules. I wanted to fit in and was hungry for ashram life. Plus, this list of rules played perfectly to my misconception that a good yogi is pure, equanimous, and perfect. It might be true, by the way, that an enlightened yogi is pure, equanimous, and perfect, but an *aspiring* yogi is impure, volatile, and imperfect, and only by realizing, accepting, and even loving that imperfection can one transform, evolve, and become free.

A few days into my stay, two close college friends, Cordelia (from my skydiving misadventures) and Carlos, visited. Cordelia was deep into her own spiritual quest of selfless service with Doctors Without Borders. Poor Cordelia's dad was forced to endure her short stints in dangerous war-torn locales. Luckily for Mr. Gallagher, though, Cordelia spent the majority of her time not in a war zone, but deep in the Amazon.*

Cordelia was not totally safe in the Amazon, either, but at least there were no tanks nearby as she paddled among the crocs, ate monkey, checked her shoes for scorpions, and worked alongside medicine men healing with shadows.

---

* Cordelia's dad, by the way, has the best and richest Boston accent I've ever heard and really demonstrates how deeply some of us have been cheated, accent-wise. While Mr. Gallagher's brogue sounds like the love child of Captain Jean-Luc Picard and *Braveheart*'s William Wallace, we New Jersians simply sound like Fran Drescher.

Like me, Cordelia lived outside the norm, so she could understand my path, my parents' worries for me, and what it felt like to not quite fit into the mainstream.

Carlos got all that too, but for a different reason. He had come out of the closet several months earlier and was adjusting to the life-altering realities that implied and allowed. Finally he could be himself. He had always suppressed so much of himself to hide his secret. As an adolescent, he had swapped musical theater for student government, and he had pretended to have crushes and had dated girls.

All that took a toll. And now he was free and trying to find his footing. When those inner voices are quelled, at first they get louder, but after enough time, they fall silent, and it takes a bit of work to wake them up. I think that's why people who have just come out often need to be so fabulous for a while. Their new identity must completely envelop and define them for a time to rekindle their inner knowing and build the trust of their inner voice that it will be heard and respected.

So Carlos, like Cordelia, understood living outside the mainstream. But neither of them understood my desire for solemn, austere monkhood. And they had not, apparently, seen the rules binder. At silent breakfast, they were giggling like chimps. At solemn morning yoga they were doing donkey kicks during downward dog. And one night, when we went for a walk after dinner and could hear the Boston Pops drifting over the lake from Tanglewood, one thing led to another and Carlos shouted, "Skinny-dip!"

Next thing I knew, they were running to the water, dropping clothes as they went. The binder is very clear on swim attire. No bikinis, no G-strings, no cutoffs; only one-piece suits for women and traditional swim trunks for men — basically, *The Great Gatsby* at the Kripalu beach. I guess Cordelia and Carlos had missed that section of the binder as well.

I was mortified but followed them in.

I had to admit that it was pretty magical under the moon, soaking in the lake, being serenaded by the Pops.

Sure enough, within minutes another group of skinny-dippers found us. They were in an energy work program and organized us all into a circle, supporting one person floating in the middle. At one point we were all standing naked, waist deep in the lake, chanting "om" and visualizing energy channeling through our hands.

As I said, the Kripalu Center was redefining itself.

Chapter 20

5:25 Am

Just throw away all thoughts of imaginary things,
and stand firm in that which you are.

— KABIR, "I Said to the Wanting-Creature inside Me"

The directors of our teacher training had scheduled as many Kripalu teachers for our morning and afternoon yoga classes as possible so that we could experience diverse teaching styles. I learned a variety of approaches to teaching breathing exercises, warm-ups, postures, guided relaxation, and meditation.

I also learned not to take people's reactions to my teaching too personally. As I watched my classmates discuss each class, I saw that yoga sometimes fires people up, and that one person might absolutely adore a teacher whom another classmate wants to skewer. People can get venomous while hating on a teacher.

I've seen yoga students display irrational loyalty toward and hero worship of their teachers. Equally, I've seen quiet, librarian-like, middle-aged yogis become rabid with anger. In holistic circles, we call this "being triggered" — something about a class triggers a strong response from a student.

Let's say a student holds a lot of tension in her lower back. Postures that focus on those muscles can tap into that tension. Sometimes a person breathes and holds the posture and moans or sobs, and the tension releases, and she feels renewed. Sometimes she says, "Whoa, that's a little too intense," and sits the pose out, as I did in Janice's yoga class at the gym in Jersey City a year earlier. But sometimes she blames the teacher for her discomfort, and a hate-fest ensues. Freud would be thrilled.

One morning our guest teacher was a tall, lean, intense fellow with a goatee who always wore a bandanna around his head. To me he looked less yoga teacher and more pirate. I think it takes a pretty intense person to have a goatee; after all, it's the worst of both facial-hair worlds — you still have to shave every day around the goatee, just like a bald-chinned person, and yet you also have to periodically trim the goatee. That's why I choose to wear the full beard.

At our 5:25 AM morning yoga practices, most teachers began with some meditation, followed by quiet chanting or breathing exercises and gentle micromovements as warm-ups. Not this fellow. A short "om," and at 5:26 we're jumping into vigorous sun salutations — not just your garden-variety *surya namaskar*, but adapted sun salutations with unexpected turns and twists and postures I had never heard of.

For example, gate posture. This was the first time I had heard of gate posture, and at 5:30 in the AM, I was in no mood. As if any rigor at all at five in the morning was not already bad enough, I actually had to pay attention to follow his directions in order to do these complex moves and postures. Which did not go so well.

My body was still half asleep and needed a gentler wake-up. In fact, I kept getting tangled up in myself, arms between legs, as if I was playing Twister after a giant shot of Novocain to each extremity.

It was just too much; I could feel my first teacher hate-fest brewing. So I lay down in relaxation posture to rest. This was not a protest. It was not really, of course, about him. It was about me, and what my body wanted — this sort of rigor so early in the morning did not feel appropriate or even healthy to me.

I was happy to be giving my body what it wanted, but I was concerned about the ramifications. To be eligible to graduate from the program, we were allowed only three class absences, and I wasn't sure if the administrator would count my lack of participation as an absence.

After the class, the administrator approached me.

"Here she comes," I thought, expecting a hard stare and a firm talking-to.

But instead, she said, "Oh, I'm so jealous that you sat that one out. I was dying to lie down, but as the class administrator, how could I?"

This was another reminder that listening and responding to my body and my intuition always pays off — a lesson I've had to learn many times. This listening to the inner voice is exactly what Kripalu teaches. It's what epitomizes, and I think distinguishes, Kripalu yoga. As Amrit said, "Your own body is the best book on yoga you will ever read."

To help you find this inner knowing and wisdom, Kripalu yoga whispers in your ear as you practice, "Relax, you're doing fine. You are already divine." That doesn't mean, "Give up" or "Be a slacker." It means, "Relax, you don't need to seek quite so fervently. You don't need to try quite so hard. There's nothing to seek outside yourself. Follow your bliss. Trust your body, trust your intuition, trust your *prana* and allow it to come forth."

That's why I opened up with Kripalu yoga. I wanted to connect with my truest self and to allow that self to manifest. Some people's true selves are hidden beneath regret, and some behind sloth or resentment. For me it was anxiety and anger. So while some folks need "Push!" or "Do it this way!" shouted in their ear to get into gear and find their truth, I needed a gentle, "Relax, don't seek quite so hard. You are already divine" to soothe the anxiety and allow the deeper me to be heard.

Chapter 21

Catharsis

Life wants us to be whole. Life wants us to remember ourselves.
Everything nudges us in that direction. The real will always triumph.

— MARION WOODMAN, in *Yoga and the Quest for the True Self*

After Amrit left and Kripalu was in a full-scale shit storm, long-time Kripalu resident Stephen Cope commented, "Well, I guess when you pray to Shiva [Indian god of transformation, also known as Shiva the Destroyer], your temple is pretty much guaranteed to burn down to the ground so that it can be rebuilt anew."

He was right. You may have seen the famous statues of Shiva as Nataraja, the dancer.* Shiva is not playing around. If you look closely, he's having his dance on the head of Apasmara Purusha, the demon of ignorance.

Shiva surely would not stand for the cotton swab delusion. He would certainly destroy the whole market, from factories to end users, and start anew. Yes, Shiva is not comfortably reclined in an easy chair reaching for the remote and a cold Sam Adams. He is crushing the head of ignorance.

---

* Shiva as Nataraja is also called Lord of the Dance, which I can't say without thinking of Irish step dancer Michael Flatley and Mike Myers's parody at the 1997 MTV Movie Awards.

So there's another distinction of Kripalu yoga. It whispers, "Relax, you're already divine," but it also says, "When you relax and nod to your internal divinity and let your emotions be free and live from your true feelings, your superficial habits and patterns and repressed feelings and blocked emotions can cleanse out (and be destroyed)."

So if you enlist full tilt in a Shiva-worshipping style of yoga in which your emotions are encouraged to come with you into class and in which people go deeply into their emotional stuff, you gotta figure it's going to come around on you one day. And sure enough, one day during yoga teacher training that summer, amid the calm Berkshire maples and oaks, my day arrived.

According to yogic philosophy we each have five *koshas*, or bodies, like layers of an onion, from the subtlest level, the bliss body, to the grossest level, the physical body. And as I mentioned earlier, according to yoga and Ayurveda, repressed emotions can become lodged as toxins in these bodies, where they can build up and cause disease.

I had healed colitis on the physical level, and now I was about to pull out the emotional roots on a deeper level. I was doing three or more hours of intense yoga every day, I was living simply and consciously, undistracted by mundane concerns, and I was in a place that invited energy to move and resolve. So after two weeks at Kripalu, I began to feel a stirring in my belly.

One morning I knew something was afoot. I went to morning yoga class as usual, but I did my own practice. I followed my intuition and the energy moving in my body, with no idea where this practice was headed. I did boat, bow, locust, cobra, sphinx, and anything else I felt guided to move into. I practiced these belly-down yoga postures with ferocious intensity, pushing hard into each posture. I usually practiced with care and gentleness, but today intensity was the call of my energy and my body.

Recall what these belly-down postures had done to me in Janice's yoga class in Jersey City a year earlier. Anytime Janice led the class into boat, bow, locust, cobra, or sphinx pose, I became very angry and would actually leave the room and return only when the class had moved on to the next group of postures, the shoulder stand series. Over time, after several months, the feelings passed. Perhaps I had strengthened my abdominal muscles, or perhaps the emotions engaging my abdomen had triggered had become safely and temporarily reburied.

Today, though, these emotions were clearly being exhumed. I flowed from posture to posture, pushing hard, and made noise and moaned and breathed into my body. I pushed my belly hard into the ground (I think to engage and activate the muscles, organs, energy, and emotions of the area). Energy was stirring and moving and beginning to swirl inside me.

After class I tried to eat breakfast, but I was too agitated. I asked a friend to sit with me outside. We talked. I was so angry, not with her, just angry. It was confusing; I had never felt anything like this before. She suggested I vent to let it out, so I did.

There, on the expansive front lawn of the Kripalu Center for Yoga and Health, overlooking the grand green valley of the Stockbridge Bowl and quiet Lake Mackinac, I started shouting nonsense, and then like Cameron in *Ferris Bueller's Day Off*, I started yelling "Fuuuuck" at the top of my lungs.

You'd think that might have disturbed some. And you're right, it did. But this type of release is not as unusual an occurrence as you might think at Kripalu, and most of the Kri-people just nodded approvingly, "Ah, he's venting. Very good." As I mentioned, Kripalu is a place of transformation, and energy often moves within people. In fact, there's an old joke at Kripalu. Someone is walking down the hall and stops to speak with a friend. "How are you?" she asks. The friend bemoans, "Terrible. I'm an emotional wreck. I have a cold. I feel like crying," to which the correct Kripalu response is, "Excellent. Keep up the good work."

When I was done with my scream-fest, I felt in no shape for class. I decided to go to the program room and fill out an absence form. I figured that instead of sitting in class, I'd walk in the woods or sleep or shout into my pillow. I knew something was moving.

In heading to the classroom, called the Kripalu Sanctuary, I wonder if I was actually reaching out for support and comforting. I went into the room and grabbed a form. The teachers and assistants were in a quiet meeting.

I can't remember falling to the ground, but the next thing I knew, I was flat on my back writhing and weeping, with no concern or holding back. It was a pure energy release; I was not crying about anything in particular, I was just weeping.

Karl, one of the assistants, came over and held my hand and offered me tissues. It was more of a sliding of the tissue box to within reach than an overt offer. Kripalu literally trains its assistants for this exact sort of experience.

Karl did not try to impede my release but offered a supportive presence, just so I knew I was not alone. He slid the tissues forward when my tears were pooling or when I needed to blow my nose. He was not telling me to stop or to pull myself together. On the contrary, he was my facilitator and pit crew as I emoted, looking out for my needs, keeping onlookers at bay. If this had gone on for days, which it never does, he would have brought out a bedpan and a sponge bath.

Karl sat with me, and I wept for quite a while.

Then I was empty, and it was all out.

Karl played by the book and supported me perfectly. He was not uncomfortable witnessing the release. He did not try to stop me or make me feel better, nor did he drag it out or dramatize it. After

I was done, he gave me a squeeze of reassurance and was ready to move on.

Which was perfect.

Another assistant, though, came over and told me that I had had a very big energy release and that I should let them know if I had any problems afterward, such as loss of hearing or vision. This, of course, freaked me out a bit.

I took a short walk and then rejoined the class. Luckily, the topic that day was meditation, so I sat in meditation on and off for three hours and let things settle and integrate. When I was done, I was filled with love and I longed for someone to share it with. I wanted someone to hug and come home to, someone with whom I could share this warmth and sweetness.

This was not exactly the same epiphany that Zach had had when he realized that he wanted to spend his life with someone. It was a bit different. I had always rejected and repressed anger. To avoid *feeling* the anger, I had navigated my life intellectually, without emotion, with my head only. That meant that I missed not only the anger but also other feelings, such as love. Today I had uncorked and dumped the anger bottle. And that allowed me to feel. It opened a door and allowed my heart to be heard. And of course the heart wants to share and connect.

This repression, by the way, was also the source of my anxiety. All true emotions — love, fear, anger, even sadness — are charged with vitality. Repressing these emotions, shutting down the heart and living from the head, denies this vitality, causing the opposite: depression and anxiety.

There was still more work to do in allowing myself to feel and express anger, and more work to do in awakening the voice of my heart, but that day they both got a few decibels louder.

After my catharsis, thankfully, I did not lose hearing or vision, though I was, for a time, able to see auras. Seriously. Or maybe it was just light residues on my retina or even a slight vision disturbance, as the assistant had warned. I actually checked a book about seeing auras (Barbara Brennen's *Hands of Light*), though, and the pictures in the book exactly confirmed what I was seeing. Either way, I didn't focus on it, and it soon subsided.

Chapter 22

Mom and Dad's

My name is George.
I'm unemployed, and I live with my parents.

— GEORGE COSTANZA, *Seinfeld*, "The Opposite," 1994

*A*fter I completed yoga teacher training at Kripalu, I moved back in with my parents. Fresh from my cathartic release, I was openhearted and reborn. But there's an old yoga joke: "If you think you're enlightened, spend a week living at your parents'."

My parents were actually wonderful, if a bit worried about my career path, but I was twenty-five and living in my childhood room, sleeping in my twin bed under my toy soldier comforter, and being called to dinner by my mom.

Now that I'm thirty-nine with my own family and all the responsibilities and stresses of making a living and being a father, some time in my old twin bed being called to dinner by my mom sounds grand, like some much-needed, sweet R & R. But back then I felt like a flop, and the whole arrangement seemed to absolutely preclude the possibility of a significant romantic relationship.

I tried to make the best of it. My yoga teaching certificate in hand, I set up a bunch of weekly classes at gyms, corporations, and churches in the area. The highlight for me was having my brother and mother as dedicated students in my Thursday evening class in the basement of a nearby church.

The force runs strong in our family, and Larry and my mom were both naturals. The day after his third class, Larry reported, "I don't know how yoga does it, but this morning I felt so open and happy and free. I felt like spinning in a field with my arms overhead and singing 'The Sound of Music.' "

But I was not totally comfortable teaching yoga. Something was wrong, and I couldn't put my finger on it. And then one day I got it.

I was in a rush heading to class. I was also hungry and didn't want to teach without eating something first. The only place I could think to stop on the way was Subway. So I parallel-parked, ran in, ordered a six-inch veggie sub, and got some water in a cup to go. I ran to the car and ate the sub while I finished the drive. Then I washed it all down with the water.

As I was pulling into the lot of the upscale gym where I was teaching that day, I realized that I was holding a large Subway Coca-Cola cup. Like a criminal hiding the smoking gun, I stashed it under my seat. That was when I realized what was wrong. I had ideas of how a yoga teacher should be, and I was not living them. The cotton swab deception was alive and well.

The problem was not that I had ideas of how I should be, or even that I was not living them, but that I was putting up an inauthentic facade as I was torn between the two. Either I needed to be a yoga teacher who did not eat fast food, or I needed to be a yoga teacher who did and was honest about it.

For me the goal of doing yoga is union, union of the internal and external parts of me, union of me with others, and union of my self with the universal all-connected self. My inauthentic facade was separating, not uniting, the two parts of me as well as separating me from others. I was putting up a false front. I could do a good perfect-yoga-teacher impression. I even had the straight posture and the bushy beard. But underneath I was conflicted and neurotic. My goal was to be honest about being human — about my crazy mind, my occasional stop at Subway, and even my guilt about the whole affair. I believe that's where growth and freedom are to be found, in transparent, compassionate, mindful honesty, at least to one's self, about one's rationales, desires, emotions, and thoughts.

I wanted to be the same Brian all the time: on the way to class and in front of the class, inside and out. So I went back to studying and took some time off from teaching. And after several more months of sleeping in my twin bed surrounded by T-ball trophies, I needed outta Dodge. I had heard that Princeton (one hour south) was a pretty hip place. So one day I hit the road and headed south on the Garden State Parkway. I had no idea what I'd find in Princeton, but on the way there, when I stopped for gas, the attendant asked me where I was headed. When I told him Princeton, he responded, "Princeton? I'm sorry for you. That place is full of hippies, commies, and faggots." I didn't feel like an argument, but now I knew I was heading to an interesting place.

Chapter 23

What Would Joshua Do?

I wish that every human life
might be pure transparent freedom.

— SIMONE DE BEAUVOIR, *The Blood of Others*

I interviewed for a room in an apartment with a few sociology grad students from Princeton University, and they offered me the spot. It was a typical large group rental in a college town, an old Victorian gone to disrepair, replete with both exquisite hand-carved moldings and vile green mold.

Complete Home Makeover would have had a field day with this place. There were beautiful Doric columns on the front porch, a stained-glass rose window in the attic, hand-carved details on the woodwork buried under fifteen coats of renters' paint, and spaces between the floorboards that offered a much unwanted and somewhat terrifying view straight down to the basement. At least this last detail made it easy to check, at any given moment, what we had in storage without having to make the treacherous trip down the swaying basement stairs.

The landlord of our house was, to put it politely, a nut job. He had grown up in one of the noisiest, most crowded cities in the world, and he shouted whenever he spoke. His words were clipped and sounded aggressive. He always sounded angry. He could be saying, "I LOVE YOU! YOU ARE WONDERFUL!" and you'd be left quivering and sobbing for your mother.

The toilet often got blocked. We'd call him and he'd show up with a plunger and, when needed, a drain snake. For those lucky enough to never encounter one, a drain snake is an indispensible but absolutely unappealing creation used to wriggle through backed-up filth and excrement to break up a clog.

After clearing the drain, our landlord would rinse his snake in the sink (which, I'm aware, sounds very randy). And when the running water would hit the drain snake, it would mix with the foul poop water on the snake and ricochet out in a three-foot radius of the sink. Mr. Tobbs thought nothing of this and would give his fingers the most superficial rinse under a trickle of water before scratching his face, rubbing his eyes, or planting a pinky deep into his ear. He was also, therefore, as you might guess, completely oblivious to my water glass and toothbrush sitting innocently on the counter, now vulnerable to the vile spray. Each time I was left with no choice but to incinerate them both.

After clearing a drain, he would deliver a short, belligerent lecture with lots of spitting. He was a women-flushing-their-tampons-down-the-toilet conspiracy theorist. He was obsessed, and no amount of reassurance from the females in the house would assuage him.

One time our toilet seat broke. He told us we were sitting on it too hard. I'm still trying to figure that one out.

I signed a lease in May and moved in for the summer with some subletters while the sociology students went their own ways for the summer. These subletters were some crazy dudes.

Nianzu, from Hong Kong, lived in the back room with his American wife. She was a master of cooking complex meals from canned food abandoned in the pantry by the previous renters. Nianzu came and went at the oddest hours, and we were all convinced that he was cheating on her. Then again, he was a nuclear physicist visiting

Princeton's elite Institute for Advanced Study, so who knows what he was really up to. Or if even she was, indeed, his wife at all. I suspect she was a fellow secret agent.

Ingvar, from Sweden, was a devout born-again Christian who was very protective of his lunch Tupperware container and spent many hours a day on the toilet, I think reading the Bible.

The third subletter was Emmanuelle, a lesbian and an architecture student finishing her degree at Princeton. She acted like I was always staring at her. She seemed to think that I had never met a lesbian before, and I'm pretty sure she believed that I had a big crush on her. Point of fact: she was *absolutely* correct on all three counts, so I couldn't really argue.

My one ray of camaraderie in the house that summer was Hugo. He was one of the sociology students who would be there for the school year. He had a very relaxed schedule that summer, and he and I hit it off. We had a great time. We'd bake bread, cook big meals, and have his friends over. We'd drink wine and play Scrabble and eat chocolate. It was very Princeton. We also built things and painted. We assembled a hammock, built shelves in the closet, painted the kitchen, and planned grand renovations. I felt very manly.

In the fall Emmanuelle, Nianzu, and Ingvar left. Hugo stayed, and the rest of the sociologists moved back in, the most interesting of whom was Joshua. Here's what you need to know about this guy: Joshua was president of the Civil Disobedience Club of Princeton University.

At first Joshua and I got off on the wrong foot. I was put off by his arrogance. But soon I realized that he was not so much arrogant as *free*. He did not play the game. He wasn't assessing what I needed to feel comfortable in every interaction. He was just himself. He listened to and followed his inner callings.

I don't mean to say that Joshua was antisocial — quite the opposite. In fact, he was one of the most charismatic people I have ever met. When people are very uncomfortable with themselves, you can feel it, and you get uncomfortable too. Joshua, in contrast, was so accepting of himself and therefore so at ease with himself in all ways, with his flaws and his strengths, that he oozed calm, and just being with him was freeing.

I'd say that my getting off on the wrong foot with Joshua really started when he hosted a party for the Civil Disobedience Club. As you might imagine, the Civil Disobedience Club attracts a certain crowd, people with names like Inferno and Epiphany and Imelda. You get the distinct sense that if you crossed these people it would not go at all well for you. And since, after all, this was Princeton, not Brown or Hampshire, where you design your own major, these disobedient folks caught me off guard.

Joshua was like special ops, like MacGyver. He could do anything he put his mind to. He could procure plutonium for the party if he really needed to. So somehow in the one hour that I was out of the house, Joshua managed to drape every wall in black sheets, block every window, and fill every room with florescent objects illuminated by black lights. I came home from yoga class to find Joshua, Inferno, Epiphany, and Imelda dancing in the Beatles' Yellow Submarine.

Joshua was not just free, he was also reckless, though that didn't matter, since he could talk his way out of anything. One time another roommate, a black belt in karate, got some bad news from a girlfriend and punched a hole in our wall. The landlord sent a maintenance guy over to fix it and told us that we'd be charged for the damage.

The maintenance guy shows up and gets to work. Twenty minutes later, sure enough, there's Joshua chatting with him in fluent Portuguese and sharing a cigarette. The guy fixed the hole, and we were never charged.

That's how it was with Joshua. He was the kind of guy who'd

register a PO box before going abroad to India and then mail himself twenty ounces of hashish.

Actually, he did that.

Though when he went to pick it up, he was convinced that there were undercover cops staking out the place, so he never went inside. That's why he'll be president one day. Anyone can mail twenty ounces of hashish from India to a PO box, but to mindfully choose to abandon it there requires real discipline.

Somehow midsemester Joshua got hold of a hydroponic growing tank. If I wanted anything more exotic or illegal than biodynamic, organically grown, fair-trade green tea, I wouldn't know where to find it.

Joshua used the tank to grow pot plants in his room. This made one of the other sociologists very nervous, and one day the cops were banging on our door. They had a search warrant and headed straight to Joshua's room. They found and confiscated his pot plants and brought him down to the station.

Most students would have been kicked out of school. Joshua talked his way out of being expelled and was only assigned community service hours. Supposedly he not only fished his plants out of the dumpster behind the police station but also, à la *Fight Club*, subversively planted marijuana seeds in the highway dividers that he was assigned to "weed" and replant as his community service.

Joshua was not perfect. I definitely don't condone his marijuana use or his flouting of the law, and thankfully a few years later he gave all that up and got into yoga and meditation. But I appreciate that he was free. And more important, he listened to his heart. When he had a crush on a girl, he did not stew in his angst but just asked her out. He used both his vastly sharp mind and his alive and alert intuition. He knew what he felt was right, and he went for it.

For years afterward, and even sometimes now, when I am unsure how to act in a new situation, I ask myself, "What would

Joshua do?" which is actually an ironic question since Joshua would never do anything just because he'd seen someone else do it; he'd do exactly what his heart, gut, and mind told him to do. So I should ask, "What do I want to do?" As they say in Buddhism, "Don't follow in the footsteps of the Buddha; seek what he sought."

I found Joshua (that's not his real name, by the way) recently on Facebook. I asked him if he was still president of a Civil Disobedience Club. He got a bit sensitive and brusquely told me that he was not, burying the subject. Then he told me that he was running for local government. That must have been why he was sensitive about the old Princeton memories.

Even though I know about Joshua's shenanigans, I'd vote for him in a heartbeat. He's free enough to make the decisions that he feels are truly right.

Plus, Joshua loves and accepts himself fully. People do bad things from self-hatred and feelings of inferiority, never from self-love. True and complete self-acceptance and self-love always arouse inspirational and moral behavior. Renowned world religions scholar Huston Smith says, in fact, that this was the very power of Jesus. He felt God's love, and in turn he was able to love his disciples so completely that their feelings of self-hatred and inferiority fell away, and in feeling this absolute love and acceptance, they became enlightened and free.

Chapter 24

ADD

You can't stop the waves, but you can learn to surf.

— SWAMI SATCHIDANANDA

That winter in Princeton, I met a psychotherapist who was trying out a new mindfulness-based therapy technique and wanted guinea pigs to work on. I would get very inexpensive therapy, and she'd get experience. At first I had said no, since I'd always (ridiculously) imagined that only pretty messed-up people went for psychotherapy, but when I bumped into her one day at the natural foods market, I thought, "Why not?" and we made an appointment.

My sessions with Valerie were sometimes triggering, sometimes calming, and always helpful. We talked about work, yoga, family, anger, love, and relationships.

Three months into our sessions, in February 1997, though Valerie knew that I'd get upset, she diagnosed me with attention deficit disorder (ADD). During the months that we had been meeting, Valerie had heard me report many common, though subtle, symptoms of ADD. I had done well throughout school, achieving excellent grades and high test scores. However, in upper grades, as school became increasingly less structured, I relied on cramming at deadlines for tests and papers. This difficulty focusing until there is urgent need, such as an imminent deadline, is a common symptom of ADD. Cramming was exhausting and very stressful, leaving me frazzled and drained.

My mind was always churning. Incessantly. To calm and relax, I drank at night, but luckily, during college, I had replaced alcohol with yoga and meditation. I used yoga to help calm and focus my mind. This is common, even in folks without ADD, but I felt reliant on, almost addicted to, yoga each day for a dose of steadiness.

After graduation, I worked as a teacher and was creative and very effective, but I found it difficult to sustain the effort all day. During my short tenure as a waiter at O'Malley's in Hoboken, I had tremendous difficulty keeping track of details while multitasking. Both these jobs left me exhausted. Thus, like many ADD people, I became an entrepreneur and started tutoring so that I could set my own hours and goals.

I demonstrated symptoms in other areas as well. In relationships, I was inconsistent. Usually, I was caring, fun, and present, but sometimes I needed to retreat and could seem aloof and disconnected. I was unpredictable and could not explain to my friends or girlfriend what was happening or why I suddenly needed space to feel sane. At home, mundane tasks exhausted me. I would lose focus after performing several in a row. The inability to multitask, or the feeling of being totally overwhelmed by several mundane tasks in sequence, is a sure sign of ADD.

Though I was successful and productive in many ways, these symptoms convinced Valerie.

Whether she was right or wrong, for a few days I was miserable about the diagnosis. I wondered if my biochemistry would limit what I could achieve. Could I work a steady job and show up consistently in a long-term relationship?

Then I remembered being diagnosed with ulcerative colitis nine years earlier. I wondered if, like colitis, ADD represented not a permanent disease or disorder but an indication that I needed to reexamine how I was living and make different choices. I began searching for evidence in holistic health literature that ADD could be treated naturally through yoga, diet, exercise, and lifestyle changes.

Finally, in an article about Ayurveda, I read that a certain imbalance can cause ADD-type symptoms. That was all it said, but it was a lead. I began researching to find how I could employ Ayurveda.

I read everything I could find on the subject. I made an appointment with a local practitioner. And in the meantime, the following weekend, at a fund-raiser for a massage school that was opening in the area, I had the opportunity to go for a fifteen-minute Ayurveda consultation with a visiting out-of-town practitioner.

Harvey, the practitioner, asked me some questions about myself and why I had come to see him. Our conversation led to the fact that I often felt cold and was bothered by the wind. He told me that my *vata dosha* was out of balance (which made sense, based on what I had learned from the Ayurvedic cookbook) and that that imbalance can show up as ADD-type symptoms. Bingo!

I asked for remediation. He made a few suggestions but didn't catch the urgency of my query. He was fixated on my sensitivity to wind, perhaps because we had only fifteen minutes together for our session, which I imagine would not have been enough time to tackle ADD.

Our conversation went something like this:

HARVEY: So you are very sensitive to wind and cold. Tell me more.

BRIAN: Ah, yeah, I don't like to be cold, and the wind bothers me.

HARVEY: Interesting...

BRIAN: What about the ADD, doc?

HARVEY: Let's stick with the wind and cold for now. This sounds like a *vata* imbalance. I recommend that every morning before you leave the house, you apply a small amount of untoasted sesame oil to every orifice of your body: lips, nostrils, ears, nipples, penis, and anus.

BRIAN: Aha.

HARVEY: Well, here's my card. Give me a call, and we can address your other questions.

And with that we were done. His eyes escorted me out, and he welcomed in his next fifteen-minute patient. I absolutely respected Ayurveda and was famished for whatever it had to teach me, but come on. Untoasted sesame oil on my nipples, penis, and anus? Was I being punked? He might as well have prescribed a pilgrimage to Coxsackie, New York.

I would have to wait until I saw the next practitioner to address my ADD, but I knew Harvey's prescription was worth a lifetime of laughs from my brother and sister-in-law. I also knew, deep down, that he was on to something with his *vata* imbalance diagnosis.

(By the way, his priceless untoasted sesame oil prescription was no different from a recommendation to use ChapStick on a windy day for dry lips. Why shouldn't the same apply for all the other "lips" of the body?)

Next I showed up for a more thorough two-hour consultation with Luther, our town's Ayurveda practitioner. Always keeping my eyes open for a meaningful occupation that could support me, I was thrilled to find a full-time practitioner. Luther seemed radiantly happy, and he made his own schedule and did meaningful work. Maybe this could be my future vocation.

But then I was at a local restaurant, a pretty elegant and healthy one, mind you, and he showed up to take my order. Imagine finding your orthopedic surgeon serving nachos for extra cash at Chili's on a Friday night. Such is often the case with holistic health. It can be done, but it's tough to make a living outside the norm, without, for example, being able to accept third-party insurance.

Luther was a man with a plan, and I always love a plan. I love taking proactive measures. He sent me home with herbs to calm my *vata* (and alleviate symptoms of ADD), Triphala powder to improve digestion and strengthen my colon, and guidelines for my daily routine: eat food cooked rather than raw, cook with a bit of oil and spice, spend quiet time every day by a lake or a gently flowing stream, avoid white sugar, look over my week's schedule every Sunday night, watch less TV, exercise, feel my feet on the ground. It was a lot less creepy than Harvey's sesame oil prescription.

Recall that Ayurveda describes three constitutions or proclivities. Everyone has his own blend of the three proclivities, and health and vitality come from respecting the needs of one's particular mix. The dominant component of my constitution, *vata dosha*, is characterized by flexibility, creativity, and spontaneity. In balance, these qualities are a joy, but in excess they manifest as ADD's spaciness, distractibility, and impulsivity.

Vata people's tendency toward flexibility and creativity can become unbounded and then look like the scatteredness of ADD. Building routine and calming the mind allow for the wonderful creativity, but without the overstimulated, overexpanded ADD state. The primary means of calming *vata* is to strengthen digestion, build routine and predictability into one's schedule, become more grounded and present in one's body, and calm the anxious mind.

Luther also suggested meditation, which can help to calm and focus the mind. It's like bench-pressing for the "muscles" of concentration.

Luther described the brain as an overgrown forest. The easiest paths to walk are the ones that are most habitually used and well worn. The same is true of the mind. That's why habits are so easy to repeat and difficult to break. If you usually reach for chocolate when stressed, that's the easiest behavior to call on in that circumstance. If your mind is used to having ten thoughts at once or losing focus after two seconds, then that is the easiest path to follow the next time as well.

Meditation practice bushwhacks new pathways of sustaining concentration, which, once worn and traveled, become new, healthier behaviors and habits. In other words, if I focus on being present rather than scattered, then over time my ability to be present improves, and it becomes easier and more natural for me to remain focused and present, until it actually becomes my default way of being.

At first, in mindfulness meditation you focus on one thing and simply practice, hopefully with loving-kindness for yourself and your imperfections, bringing attention back to the point of focus whenever you notice that your mind has wandered. Whether it wanders to the pasta fra diavolo you had for lunch, the TPS report that Bill at work keeps nagging you about, or a fight you just had with your spouse, each time you notice this happening, you can gently return the mind to your point of focus.

The breath is a terrific point of focus. It is a steady internal metronome that I use to ground myself. So for mindfulness meditation, you can focus on the sound and sensations of breath coming into and going out of your body.

You can focus on the sensations of your philtrum (don't worry, this is not a naughty bit; your philtrum is the indentation below your nostrils and above your lips) as air passes by, or you can focus on the rise and fall of the abdomen with each breath. To help you stay focused, you can even count breaths from one to ten. If your mind wanders, and you lose track before ten, no problem. Whenever you realize that you have wandered, simply relax and start over again at one. And if you are already a Zen master or a Jedi and can actually make it to ten, then simply start over again at one.

Eventually the pathways in the mind of distraction, of being pulled away from the moment or from a task, become grown over. And the practice bushwhacks and fortifies pathways in the brain that allow a formerly distractible ADD person to stay focused, to maintain concentration, not just when something is very interesting, but at will.

Even before Luther's meditation prescription, I had already been practicing this regularly, ever since Yolanthe's yoga classes in Hoboken. And it was indeed helping me not only during meditation practice but somewhat in my day-to-day life as well.

But I wanted to feel even more focused, even less scattered and distractible. In my daily life my mind was still in many places at once. I'd be washing soap off my armpits in the shower and thinking about asking out Bernice at the health food store. Or worse, I'd be thinking about Bernice and forget to wash off the soap and then wonder two hours later why my armpits itched like a motherfuncher.

This explained why I, like all ADD sufferers and, really, like most scattered Americans, had to routinely check if I had locked my car door. Sometimes I was not present for interactions and afterward I'd feel insecure, wondering, "How did that go? Did I say anything stupid?" Sometimes I literally couldn't remember.

I devised a plan. I would be there for my interactions and activities throughout the day. *All day* would be a meditation. I would focus entirely on whatever I was doing at any given moment. Then I wouldn't have to wonder, later, whether I had locked the front door, turned off the oven, or said the right thing to Jenny, because I'd have been right there and I'd be able to remember all of it.

This was certainly my best experiment yet. I would actually pause as I locked a door so that I was present and so that later I'd remember I had done it. I would rein in my mind and be in my body as I walked along the river, washed the dishes, and chatted with people. It took lots of effort, lots of reminders — I literally wore strings on my fingers and made signs to post on my bathroom mirror and my bedroom door — but it worked. I was like a monk. And with time I was more focused and more present for more of my day.

Which brings us to our fifth Key to Happiness. Put simply,

Meditate.

It's the bomb. I know of nothing else that is as unequivocally effective and transformational. It's relaxing and helps you focus. It raises your level of consciousness, clarifies your mission, and makes it easier to identify and follow your bliss and intuition.

You should meditate. Really. I'll only say this once, and then I'll drop it so that I won't seem a nudge. But, really, meditate (and if you already meditate, meditate *more*). You can check out some basic instructions in appendix 3.

༄

That day in Princeton Luther also mentioned that he had studied Ayurveda at the New England Institute of Ayurvedic Medicine in Massachusetts, and that a person could get a master's degree in holistic studies through the independent studies program at Lesley College in Cambridge.

I was intrigued. This might allow me to take my career to the next level, satisfy my family's calls for a higher degree, and study yoga and Ayurveda full-time. I looked into it and decided to put together an independent study proposal. My plan would include a nine-hundred-hour Ayurveda program with the New England Institute of Ayurvedic Medicine, programs at Kripalu, a meditation retreat, and lots more.

A few weeks later I was accepted to the program, and my study plan was approved.

In April I drove from Princeton to Porter Square in Cambridge for the first of ten weekend Ayurveda courses, and in May, I packed up my stuff in Princeton, said good-bye to the sociologists, and headed to a monthlong holistic health teacher training program at Kripalu. I figured after HHTT I'd move to Northampton, Massachusetts. A famous yogi lived there, and I'd heard that he was looking for a few very serious students. Me, please!

Chapter 25

Shaktipat

Be mindful what you ask for. You might actually get it.

— Unknown

It had been two years since my yoga teacher training at Kripalu, and I was glad to be back: yoga at 5:30 AM, silent mindful breakfast, inspiring classes, healthy food, more yoga, and bed at 9:30 PM.

Being at Kripalu was easy for me — I could meditate, process, and eat mindfully all day, but multitasking laundry and finding the envelope that came with my gas bill was much, much harder. In fact, most of my ADD/*vata* triggers were mundane daily logistics. Answering the phone while opening my mail or putting away groceries while having a conversation could leave me fried.

At Kripalu these logistical tasks were unnecessary, and, ever since Oskar's class in Georgetown, I had been at home and in my element in any yoga environment. So at Kripalu I felt like a spiritual superhero.

High on this trip, I was meditating one day in Swami Kripalu's special meditation room, and I was feeling particularly empowered and inspired and connected to Swami Kripalu's ubiquitous energy in the place. Staring at his photo on the altar, I said, "I'm ready. I'm ready for the next step."

There was definitely a cocky, "Bring it" energy to my claim, which is probably pretty good evidence that I was not, in fact, ready. And in fact, I received a clear response to my challenge. In my mind I heard, "(*gentle, loving chuckle*) You're not ready. Go into the forest and get grounded."

I heard the admonition, acknowledged it, and mindfully chose to ignore it. "I hear you," I said, "but I think I'm ready. Bring it."

Was I Luke flouting Yoda's grandmotherly warnings not to follow the calls of Han Solo? Luke's impertinence was part of his Jedi coming-of-age, part of his becoming a man-Jedi. What about me? Was I showing the necessary independence in the process of becoming a man-Jedi-yogi, or was I a fool?

And the correct answer is...I was a fool.

Lunch break ended, and I went back to class. That afternoon's topic was energy work. At the end of the session, the teacher asked if anyone had announcements. Sure enough, one of the older students in class, an odd, somewhat antisocial woman named Genevieve, came up to the front and said something like, "I am a spiritual teacher, and I'm looking for a new student, if anyone is interested."

In hindsight, I'm surprised the program facilitators did not step in and have her removed from the grounds right then and there. But at the time, all I thought was, "Whoa, Swami Kripalu came through fast."

After class I went over and asked to become her student.

We went to a corner of the room and set to work immediately. I had never paid much attention to this woman before. Now that I looked at her, she seemed in pain, her face contorted and her shoulders a bit hunched. She also seemed half present, like a medium receiving constant mental transmissions from the beyond. She was pretty odd, really, but I was not put off. What can one expect when asking to be taken outside the ordinary matrix of reality? Plus, she was exactly how I'd imagined the one-eyed, warted, madwoman-shaman who lived at the edge of town (and perhaps the edge of reality).

Genevieve told me the protocol for our meetings. When we met, we would greet each other with a bow, and then we would sit together quietly for a few moments. We did that.

She told me that, alternately, we could begin by hugging, but she assured me that we would never need to sleep together. I nodded, said, "Okay," and smiled, as though to say, "Glad we cleared that one up," but inside, of course, I was thinking, "WTF!? That's pretty creepy. Why even mention that?"

She continued, "Tell me a bit about yourself." I did. And then Swami justice hit, and it was brisk and severe. Genevieve stared into my eyes and said, "You know who you really are, right?"

With her words, something went pop at the base of my spine. Energy shot up my spinal column, and I was crying. I felt joy and bliss. It was Jerry Garcia's green light but turned up way too high. As the energy traveled up my spine, I was losing myself, and I couldn't handle it. I clamped down tight and shut it off.

All this took only a few seconds.

The energy traveling up my spine had reached my heart when I shut it off. The bliss faded, and I was a wreck, like Lot's wife having glanced back at Sodom, like the guy who glanced at the open ark in the first *Indian Jones* movie.

This experience of energy being released at the base of the spine and traveling up, filling a person with bliss, is called *shaktipat*. According to yogic tradition, *shaktipat* is initiated by a guru's touch either literally in person or figuratively from a distance, or even through the touch of a disciple. *Shaktipat* is said to be a quickening, a drastic awakening of transformative spiritual energy in the recipient. As Elizabeth Gilbert writes in *Eat, Pray, Love*, "After that touch, the student might still labor for years [I would add "or lifetimes"] toward enlightenment, but the journey has at least begun. The energy has been freed."

My *shaktipat* experience had seemed to go very wrong.

It made sense that the energy had stopped rising at my heart area. That was an area that needed work. It had received a tune-up, and its hinges had been oiled during my yoga teacher training catharsis, but my head still ruled the roost, keeping my heart cobwebbed and in storage.

After my very short visit with Genevieve, a tornado of energy was swirling in my heart area. I recall walking down the long driveway of Kripalu the following day and feeling, almost seeing, the small tornado of energy swirling just in front of my chest. I was an emotional mess. I was not upset about anything that I could name; I was just shaken, disturbed, and stirred up.

I had gotten exactly what I had asked for, and I wasn't ready for it. That experience sent me right into the woods for grounding and comfort. I have always found sitting with trees to be very calming, and I spent every minute that I could, for the rest of that month, sitting among the trees in the forest.

Chapter 26

Urine Therapy Virgin

We need to respect the fact that it is possible to know
without knowing why we know and accept that
— sometimes — we're better off that way.

— MALCOLM GLADWELL, *Blink*

During holistic health teacher training, on a day off from classes, I traveled to Northampton with two friends, La and Emily. They wanted some R & R in the "big city," and I wanted to find an apartment. La and Emily went off to do some shopping at the natural foods store, while I looked for a newspaper.

Back then Northampton's *Daily Hampshire Gazette* was one of the few remaining afternoon-release newspapers in the country. So when the paper came out, I ran off to a pay phone and started making calls.

I was using a phone in the back of a store, when suddenly I was overcome by the overpowering stench of human feces. I don't know if you've ever smelled human feces without the buffer of toilet water, but it puts dog poop to shame. Human poop makes you want to spread dog poop on a saltine.

I looked around and saw on the floor next to me, right there in the store, a steaming load. Seeing the pile, it clicked in my mind that as I had been speaking to the landlord, I noticed out of the corner of my eye that someone was urgently headed to the bathroom next to the pay phone, but that when they pulled the handle, it was locked. I suppose they had to go badly, because they must have dropped drawers and let loose. Somehow, while speaking to landlords, I had missed that critical part not two feet from my feet.

I was now alone with a steaming pile. Overcome by the stench and wary of being fingered as the culprit, I panicked, dropped the phone, and fled.

It's no surprise that this event went down in the store's lore, and eight years later when I became friends with the manager, he remembered it and said, "Holy shit, you were there, you saw the guy who did it? Yeah, that poop-and-run is famous. I was the newest employee then, so I had to clean it up!"

I can't really blame that poop-and-run, since it only cost me one landlord, but I did not secure an apartment that day. I had a vision for the apartment I wanted. I had spent many years sharing apartments with cockroaches and mold and was ready for the next level. I wanted clean and quiet. I wanted some nature. I wanted peace, a place where I could meditate and practice yoga. A place to untie my knots. In my kitchen I wanted to set up a rice cooker and a blender for making almond milk, and I wanted to buy a slotted spoon for poaching eggs. No more mac 'n' cheese and ramen noodles.

Finally, a few weeks later an apartment came through, and it was perfect. I had called the number in the ad, and the message said, "Hi, you've reached David. This Saturday's 9:15 AM yoga class will be held outdoors in Pulaski Park. Please leave a message. Thanks."

I left a message with my usual spiel, "clean and quiet," and added that I had just moved to Northampton from a month at Kripalu. I got a call back instantly. David was the landlord and also the owner of the Northampton Yoga Center, so he loved that I was a yoga teacher.

I went to see the place, a converted attic. It was cute, very clean, and on a very quiet street. There was even a trailhead nearby that led into the woods and to a swimming hole. David, who owned the place, lived on the first floor. He was a sweet guy and a fellow yogi.

I owned only clothes and a few books. My most expensive possessions were my three-season sleeping bag and a gold Georgetown watch that my parents had given me at graduation. I had no bed, no bookshelf, and no pots or pans. So I went to a few stores and maxed out my credit cards.

I moved in. I knew literally no one in Northampton. I spent my days writing my independent studies master's thesis, hiking in the woods, doing yoga, and setting up my tutoring practice. I was happy to be living so simply and intentionally, but I was also tremendously lonely.

I also had no TV, and I now understood how the settlers three hundred years ago had time to churn butter. Without three hours a day of *Seinfeld* and *Cheers* there would have been time enough to bake my own bread and then churn the butter to go with it.

In continuing with my anti-ADD regimen, I did one thing at a time. I was deliberate. I was mindful. I concentrated on bringing awareness into my body. All day was a meditation. "I am mindful that I am washing my hands. My hands feel wet. I am drying my hands. My hands feel dry. I am walking. I feel my feet on the ground." I was inside a *Dick and Jane* book, and I was the narrator.

I had no shower, so I took baths out of the antique iron claw-foot tub that someone, in a feat of strength and genius, had gotten up to the attic bathroom.

I did have two social salvations every month. Once a month I would head back to Kripalu to meet my teacher for a mentoring session. I'd see him and bump into old friends, maybe even have lunch with someone. And one weekend each month I would make the two-hour drive to Cambridge for my Ayurveda class. I had made a small circle of friends there. The classes were not very interactive, and mostly I sat and took notes, but my friends and I would have lunch and sometimes dinner together.

People in the Ayurveda program saw me as a monk. I was impressed with their involved, successful lives, and they were impressed with my attention and intention. Unlike people immersed in the world with too much to do, I did one thing at a time and I did it with my full attention. I was not juggling work and kids. I was not bucking for a promotion or networking to make connections.

I was determined to do all I could to balance my *vata*. So as I learned additional Ayurvedic recommendations to balance *vata*, I applied that learning. I ate only *vata*-balancing foods. I performed sesame oil massage every day before I bathed. I did gentle yoga, relaxation, and meditation. I slept eight or nine hours a night. I spent at least one hour every day sitting next to a large tree on the bank of the gently flowing Mill River. I never rushed. I drank a daily *vata*-balancing tonic of warm milk, sprouted almonds, cardamom, and honey. I even considered using the *vata*-balancer's ultimate weapon — sesame oil enemas.

After six months of this, I was much more grounded and focused, and my digestion was strong. I had surely balanced my *vata*, but I had gone too far. In eating only cooked foods with lots of oil and spices, I had balanced my *vata*, but I had also aggravated the *pitta* in my constitution. *Pitta* is the element of fire, responsible for intensity. I had become very intense, though I didn't realize it as it was happening.

A woman cleaned my landlord's house every month. I was there one day while she was cleaning, and she was visibly uncomfortable.

"Why?" I asked.

"You're a bit intense," she said. "You must realize it?"

What did she mean? Sure, I was staring her down from only two feet away as she chose which sponge to use. Sure, I appraised and second-guessed her every decision. Who wouldn't?

Alas, she was right. I was way too intense. I even had other *pitta* imbalance symptoms. Since *pitta* is the energy of fire, a *pitta* imbalance shows up fiery and hot: as intensity, anger, skin rash, and acid stomach. I did not have any overflowing anger that I was aware of, although in my isolated, monkish Northampton existence, I hardly interacted with anyone whom I could get mad at, and my ability to feel and express anger was still pretty blocked anyway.

But I had one heck of an angry rash on my back. Until then I had not made the connection that it was a *pitta* imbalance, that it was the result of my incredibly dedicated and extreme *vata*-balancing regimen. I was embarrassed as hell by the rash. Its only upside was that it gave me excellent fodder for allowing my spiritually inconvenient ego to be crushed.

One month when my rash was at its worst, I was at a weekend Ayurveda training and we were having a rare interactive class. A doctor had been flown in from India to teach us an Ayurvedic cleansing massage called Swedna. Students were divided into groups of four. One student would be the patient, and the others would practice the massage. I was terrified of being chosen as a patient and having to expose my rash. The class began, and I was immediately picked. Reluctantly, I took off my shirt and lay facedown on the massage table.

I enjoyed the treatment as much as my ego would allow. I was unaware, however, that as soon as the teacher saw the blazing condition of my back, he, of course, chose me to be in front of the entire class for his next treatment. Facedown on the table, I was wheeled around and shuffled about and then asked to sit up, only to realize that my angry, rashed-out back was on display for all eighty-nine students and teachers in the class.

I was mortified as the teacher demonstrated the treatment.

Of course, no one was driven from the room by the sight of my back, as I had feared they would be. In fact, everyone was enthralled. These were students studying Ayurveda, eighty-five soon-to-be holistic healers. In a room full of dermatologists, I would have gotten eighty-two cortisone recommendations and perhaps three calendula suggestions from the more holistic Boulder and Asheville doctors, but here, in Ayurveda school, I received some...other advice.

"Try urine therapy," one very clear-skinned couple told me. "Cured his eczema," the woman encouraged. They told me to catch half a cup midstream from my first pee of the day. A warm morning cocktail.

Another well-meaning classmate recommended standing on my head forty-five minutes a day, and another recommended taking red clover and milk thistle to clean out my blood and liver.

One more recommendation stands out. I am not lying when I tell you that one man actually recommended applying leeches. And he was not from a time capsule or the 1978 Steve Martin "Theodoric, Barber of York" *Saturday Night Live* skit.* In fact, leeches are a highly respected, though now little used, Ayurvedic treatment. Since *pitta* is associated with the blood, a *pitta* imbalance can be treated by a good bloodletting, which allows the body to make new, healthier blood. We modern folks, especially men, are all at a severe disadvantage, since leeches make us think of the swamp scene in *Stand by Me*. At the mere mention of Gordie having to reach into his tightie-whities to peel off that obese and bloody leech, any man who has seen this movie will immediately wince and twist his legs.

I was the pet project of the group — just what I needed to cure my fear of exposing my rash. The group was definitely not horrified, and instead I was a celebrity for the weekend.

I appreciated the suggestions, though it was actually my teacher at Kripalu a few weeks later who cracked the rash code. He said,

---

* "Why, just fifty years ago, they thought a disease like your daughter's was caused by demonic possession or witchcraft. But nowadays we know that Isabelle is suffering from an imbalance of bodily humors, perhaps caused by a toad or a small dwarf living in her stomach."

"Hmm, so you slather sesame oil all over your back every day, and then you sit in warm bath water, and you don't ever shower off. Maybe you should lay off the oil for a bit and even hook up a shower attachment to the tub faucet." Simple. Elegant. Genius. It worked. A few weeks later my back was clean and clear, and I was still a urine therapy virgin.

That rash made me realize that I had overdone it. I eased back on the *vata* management. I started eating salads and less oil and spice. My six-month *vata*-balancing intensive had paid off, though. I was still creative, but more focused, more grounded, and less distractible. I still had the proclivity for ADD symptoms, and had to watch my *vata*, but I did not present with ADD anymore. It was the same with colitis. I imagine that I still had the latent potential for colitis if, say, I lived as I used to (without exercise, always stressed, no fiber, holding in emotions), but I had passed my two-year period and was blessedly colitis free.

⁂

In Northampton I wanted to continue the work I had begun with my Princeton psychotherapist, Valerie. So I consulted the local holistic magazine *Many Hands*, with its vast directory of holistic practitioners. I paged through looking for a psychotherapist with a mindfulness bent and found a woman who advertised to include in her sessions not only meditation but also Ayurveda. I called and set up an appointment.

The following Tuesday at the designated time, I drove to the address she gave me. I found the door and went into the waiting room.

The waiting room was homey and very comfortable, if a bit messy. There was a sofa, a few chairs, and a coffee table with magazines and a few novels. There was also a half-full cup of tea on a saucer with a half-eaten English muffin. And oddly, on the carpet, someone had left behind a pair of woolen socks. Keep in mind that when you live in Northampton, Massachusetts, hometown of Augusten Burroughs's *Running with Scissors*, this is of particular concern.

I flipped through a copy of *Natural Health* magazine as I waited. That's when the therapist, whom I immediately recognized from her photo in *Many Hands*, walked through the waiting room. Topless.

Two years earlier, at Ruby's massage parlor in High Point, I was proud to have been so naive and pure. This time I was pissed. "How could I have missed this again!?" I felt like knocking my head like Will Ferrell in *Old School*: "Dang it! I'm such an *idiot*!"

My "therapist" was wearing a towel around her waist and nothing on top. Her hair was wet. She ignored me completely as she passed through, all business. She went through to her office, did not shut the door, dropped her towel, and put on her panties, as I watched and waited.

I could see past her, into the rest of her office, and plain as day, there was a big bed. It was not red velvet, mind you, it was more respectable than that, but it was still a bed in my naked psychotherapist's office.

The possibilities raced through my mind:

1. Sex therapist? It didn't mention that in *Many Hands*.
2. Some funky Ayurveda connection? One of the seven branches of Ayurvedic medicine is dedicated wholly to fertility, after all. No. Ayurveda may have remedies for fertility, and it may recommend employing nontoasted sesame oil on one's penis and anus to protect against the wind, and it may advise the use of vomit therapy or even leeches on occasion, but I had not yet heard

of Ayurvedic sex therapists, at least not in the United States.

3. Maybe she's just a free spirit. What do clothes matter, anyway? We're all really just animals when it comes down to it. Maybe it frees up her clients. Makes them feel safe to be vulnerable when she herself has been so vulnerable and naked. This is Northampton, after all. In fact, I once heard of a totally legit, nonsexual, therapeutic massage style that was performed with both the client and the therapist naked. It was said to free up the energy and set everyone more at ease.

4. And I considered the only other option: Prostitute? Maybe...

Then, as in a Hitchcock film when the protagonist has a revelation and is shaken to the core with the whole frame spinning out of control, I suddenly realized that this was *not*, in fact, her office, and I was *not*, in fact, in a waiting room.

I was sitting, unbeknownst to her, in her den, and I had just watched her walk, naked, from the shower to the bedroom in her own private apartment. Her office had another entrance a few yards away from this one, which I now remembered seeing in the parking lot.

I was a Peeping Tom. She was getting ready for work, and as in a porn shop viewing booth, I had just watched her put on her panties. I was mortified.

I considered my options:

A. Approach her bedroom and fess up to what just happened. Maybe we'd share a hearty laugh.

No way. Much, much too creepy. She'd scream. She'd freak out. She'd call the cops.

B. I could quietly put down my magazine, stand up without making the sofa creak, tiptoe across the floor, and ease out the door to head for the other entrance, where there were likely to be no naked people.

I chose option B. There was a risk, though. Turning myself in would be better than getting caught as I fled the scene. Still, I went with B.

I made it out quietly and reentered the building through the correct door.

A few minutes later, she appeared, fully dressed, and quite smartly at that, to welcome me in.

During the hour, we talked about my lack of friendships in town. And she never knew that I had seen her naked, that I knew she wore daisy panties.

Probably for the best.

I'm wondering now, though, fifteen years later, whether she'll read this book and piece it all together.

Chapter 27

Silence

Don't just do something, sit there.

— SYLVIA BOORSTEIN[*]

*A*few weeks after my naked therapy session, I was headed to the next installment of my independent study, a three-day intensive meditation retreat at the Insight Meditation Society in Barre, Massachusetts. I drove for an hour through winding small-town roads, around the giant Quabbin Reservoir, and into sleepy Barre.

I checked in and was shown to my "bedroom." IMS is famous for its austerities, so when I say bedroom, this is very generous and even metaphorical. My bed had as much to do with that big jobber you bought at Sleepy's as my sons' couch-cushion fort does with your actual house. My bed was a two-inch-thick egg crate foam pad — not the high-tech camping sort — and it was laid out on top of a few slats of wood.

Why such austerity? Was this some sort of S and M camp? No.

---

[*] I'm not sure that Sylvia actually coined this phrase, but she has authored a book by that name, so I figure she's as relevant a source as anyone. Plus, she is a wonderful and very funny meditation instructor. I also especially like the title of her book *That's Funny, You Don't Look Buddhist.*

A dash of austerity and simplicity on a meditation retreat turns up the noise of the mind as it bitches about things so you can hear it more clearly. It's not masochistic, it's just that an uncomfortable bed brings up fears and mild aches and pains and allows you to experience your body more clearly. Or maybe if I had seen the beds in other group rooms (which I never did, since no one speaks or interacts for the entire retreat), I would have realized that my accommodations were punishment for paying the bottom end of the workshop's sliding scale.

After I settled my stuff into my small parcel of the group room, I headed to the first meditation sit. The teacher introduced himself and welcomed us, and we were off and running. Or sitting, as the case may be.

We sat quietly for our first forty-five-minute meditation segment. No problem. I am the mac daddy of meditation, the godfather of good sitting; wait till these other chumps behold the glory of my practice.

I was unconscious of its ramifications and its significance, but that really was the basic tenor of my thoughts. My ego was definitely invested in Brian Leaf as an accomplished meditator.

I find consistently that that sort of arrogance, like what I had shown at Kripalu before my *shaktipat* experience with Genevieve, invites trouble. In fact, that's the whole point of the austerity and of the sitting together: to expose the noise of the mind, and to expose imperfections. Not so we can berate, bemoan, or even correct them, but so we can notice and perhaps forgive, allow, and even love them.

Lots of things can turn up the noise of the mind at a meditation retreat. There's the lack of distraction: no phone calls, no checking messages, no Internet, no TV, no chocolate, no speaking. Just you and your body and mind.

And then there's the food. Actually the food, at least for the uninitiated, seems a cruel joke. My sister and I refer to it simply as fart food. You're sitting all day in a great big room with three hundred people who are eating only beans, rice, and dry crackers for lunch. Plus, it is very difficult to sculpt exciting, sensual food fantasies from your meditation cushion when beans, rice, and dry crackers are all you have to look forward to. And, again, that's the whole point — no distractions, just you and your body and mind.

At home I sat in meditation every day, twice a day, for thirty or forty minutes. But between those morning and evening sits, I washed and dressed and ate and worked and studied and went hiking and paid bills and did the dishes and watched movies and read books and, on a good day, even had sex.

But here, on retreat, between those two polar sits were just countless other meditations. And with no diversions or escapes, since neither the dining hall nor my bedroom offered any splurges or luxuries to look forward to. That turns up the volume of the mind big-time. And behind every arrogance lurks a deep insecurity knocking to get out. So while for a few sits I was in my element and on top of the world, soon I was a suffering, insecure wreck.

On day one of the meditation retreat, my ego held strong — at first. Then, toward evening, I started coming undone, namely about a guy sitting behind me. I saw this guy only in rare over-my-shoulder glances or when we were getting up or sitting down. He seemed very confident.

My back was beginning to get sore from sitting so straight for so long, and yet somehow he still sat straight as an arrow. By the second sit of the evening, I was in agony. And he seemed placid and at ease. From twenty-five inches behind me, he watched me suffer. And worst of all, he knew that he was better than me.

"You're not better than me!" I thought-yelled at him.

In my mind through the next day and a half we fought epic *Lord of the Rings* battles. He was the evil force of the watching eye, and I was the oppressed force of good. I really hated this guy, or, more precisely, I resented his smugness and the way that he patronized and judged me.

I could feel his gaze on the back of my head. He saw when I slumped, and I could imagine his sanctimonious half-smile of victory. I was so angry at this guy I wanted to scream.

On the last day, during a particularly long sit and after a particularly vicious fight between the two of us in my mind, I turned my head to peek at him to see if he was still sitting tall, and...he was gone.

Who knows how long he had been gone for.

You learn a lot about yourself and the way you think at a meditation retreat. Most likely this guy had barely noticed me, and I can't imagine he gave a poop as to how or even if I sat in meditation. To him I was a head of hair about twenty-five inches away for almost three days. Nothing more.

It had never been he who was judging me so harshly.

Of course it had always been *me*.

The three days over, I went to my parcel of a room and packed up my things. I did not feel nearly as high-and-mighty or arrogant. It didn't seem to matter so much anymore how straight my sitting posture was.

The retreat was a success.

Obviously, the goal of meditation is not to sit perfectly but to become more aware of what one's silly mind is doing. Instead of *being* it, we see it, and are therefore separate from it. We are freer from its silliness. We identify ourselves as the thinker, not as the thoughts. In seeing my battles with that guy, I could walk away less judgmental, more tolerant, and more loving of myself and of others.

I loaded up my car and headed home. I enjoyed my cushy bucket seat. I enjoyed Elton John and Phish on the radio, and I looked forward to my apartment and my soft bed. I stopped along the way for a few slices of pizza. I had earned a little comfort.

Chapter 28

My Anger Mattress

*A*fter the meditation retreat I was back to my monkish life in Northampton. Though I did not sit in meditation for hours a day or sleep on a wafer-thin mattress, I was pretty silent and mindful and basically living a retreat. I was learning a lot, but I was also still very lonely and desperate for social interaction. So when the time came to head to Kripalu for a monthlong massage training, I was thrilled. In early June I locked up my Northampton apartment and set off for some social interaction in the Berkshires.

At Kripalu I was assigned to a small dorm room with seven other guys, all students in the monthlong program. Does Kripalu draw unusual folks, or is everyone unusual when you share their room, watch their morning routine, and really get to know them?

Marty was a pragmatist. He knew life at Kripalu well enough that he had packed a hospital-grade urine receptacle. He had a top bunk and knew that waking up in the middle of the night to pee meant getting down from the bunk, attempting not to wake anyone on the creaky bunk ladder, opening the squeaky door, walking down the long hallway to the men's bathroom, and then repeating all that on the way back. This long process and the focus it takes to keep it quiet can leave a person wide awake at three in the morning. Thus, his urine receptacle. So every now and then during the month, I'd awake at night to a sound, and think, "What in the world is that sound?" Then I'd realize, "Oh, that's Marty peeing into his urine receptacle, right there in his bed." And I'd think, "Brilliant!" and fall back to sleep.

I had a different solution, by the way, to the Kripalu midnight pee problem. I drank lots of water in the morning and early afternoon, and then, like Bart Simpson's Grampa, I simply didn't consume any fluids for a designated amount of time before bed. This was three hours for me, though I think it's more like nine for Grampa Abe.

The second most interesting member of the dorm was Fabio, a bartender and native of the Bahamas who worked in hotels. He wanted to switch from tending bar to giving poolside massage. Really, he was a pretty normal guy, but throw the name Fabio and a Bahamian accent on anyone, and suddenly he is exotic, fascinating, and hilarious.

The most interesting, and by that I mean the most disturbing, was Pavak. He was way too excited about the fact that the training had only eight guys and twenty-eight women. I know this because he would say things like, "I want to massage all twenty-eight women in the group! I hope I get assigned a hot mama today!" And his Indian accent made this somehow even creepier, probably because at a yoga ashram one expects something said in an Indian accent to come from the master and to uncover the mysteries of the universe rather than to be a comment on Jenny's hot abs. Apparently, or so he said, he was a tantric master and could sustain erection and postpone orgasm for days. Ultimately, he got kicked out of the program.

So with Marty, Fabio, Pavak, and a few garden-variety Kri-people, I spent a lovely month.

After graduation, even though I worked only briefly as a professional massage therapist, I did get my massage license in Northampton. Interestingly, a massage license in Northampton still fell under the category "the giving of vapor baths," a throwback, I suspect, to the popularity of Turkish baths in the 1900s. To me this seemed a little too close to Ruby's outfit, though all those years later I knew she'd be proud of me.

After the bodywork training, I was offered a temporary position working at a yoga center in Montclair, New Jersey. I was hungry for community and, anyway, I wanted experience running a small center to see whether I might eventually want to open such a place myself.

The yoga center in Montclair was interesting for two reasons. First, this was the height of the tech boom, and everyone in New Jersey traded stocks. If you invested in technology companies you made money. I had not planned to trade; in fact, a few weeks earlier I would have considered it beneath me. But at a party a friend recommended a stock. I bought it and made $2,000. I thought, "Wow, that was nice," and I started trading too.

Literally everyone I knew in New Jersey traded. My piano teacher traded. We'd exchange stock tips at lessons. He'd get tips from his personal trainer at the gym, a big, hairy guy named Sal, who'd say, "Jim, ya dumb bastard, if you don't buy [such and such stock], I'm gonna kill you 'cuz you're so dumb."

Trading fever was omnipresent. I'd go for a massage, and my massage therapist and I would exchange tips — of course she was a former Wall Street hedge funder turned massage therapist.

The funniest stock trader was my boss at the yoga center. He traded daily. And he bought absolute crap stocks, the kind that cost four cents and whose companies promise to go to four dollars once they find gold in the hills or go live with their new website.

We'd serenely register clients for a yoga class, sign them in, punch membership cards, make announcements, walk mindfully out of the room, and then, once out of sight, literally sprint into the back room to watch the stock ticker and yell at our brokers. It was actually a great time. I guess we were not the only ones, because I'm told that eTrade had a commercial parodying this scenario exactly.

My trader turned massage therapist called the situation, though. She said, "When everyone is trading, it's time to bail out." I thought this was a bit elitist, but I see now that she didn't mean it that way. She just meant that when everyone is trading, prices are driven up, and there's a bubble. She was right, and pretty soon the bubble burst.

The other interesting thing about the yoga center was that like nearly all owners of yoga centers and health food stores and new age shops, the owners of my center were absolutely batty. You might expect these folks to be evolved and conscious, and maybe they are, but always, without fail, they are also quite loopy. My bosses were no exception to the rule. Again, I suppose, when one is deeply committed to seeing things as they truly are and to stepping, if necessary, outside the ordinary matrix of habitual reality, things can get pretty wild.

That year in Montclair it also became increasingly clear to me that I had difficulty feeling anger. Zach had actually informed me of this on our trip, and that had pissed me off to no end, but I only experienced that anger as a vague feeling of tension and frustration. I realized that the channel in my body/mind for feeling anger was blocked. When I was angry, I would just feel uncomfortable and not know why.

Recall that at Kripalu, during yoga teacher training, I had dumped twenty years of stored angst in a fit of catharsis. Now I saw that it was backing up again, and I needed to learn to deal with anger in the moment, not just dump it every two decades.

My teacher at Kripalu gave me a homeopathic to clear the block and said that it would not make me any angrier per say, but that it would break through the block, allow the anger into my consciousness, and force me to deal with it.

I took the one-time homeopathic dose in his office and headed home. Then things started to heat up.

Previously, the feedback loop of realizing I was angry and of then expressing that anger was totally blocked. I was not totally serene, mind you; I was just passive-aggressive. So with the homeopathic stewing in my system I went about my days. But now, when something made me mad, I'd realize, not right away, but soon after. At first this sensation was unfamiliar: What was this uncomfortable feeling in my stomach and chest? Ah, anger.

At first I did nothing about this feeling, but then it grew, and grew, and bothered me, and grew — blast this darned homeopathic — until I had to do something about it. I must have seemed like a freak. I'd call people — sometimes total strangers — three days later and say, "Remember three days ago when you sold ten slices of Swiss cheese to a guy wearing a blue jacket? Yeah, well, that was me, and you said I looked too thin. That made me very angry!"

I called massage therapists, dentists, store clerks, my father, my sister, my yoga teacher. I felt like a menace. But I knew I had to keep calling until the feedback loop in my body was quicker, until I would get angry, know it right away, and act then and there. I also knew that once I could do that, I could choose whether or not to act out the anger, but that now, as an anger novitiate, I had to act on it every time. I could not trust the voice in my head that said, "Ah, come on, no biggie, let it go." That voice was the one that I had used until now to repress my anger, and it was not to be trusted. Later I could make the choice from a free place, not from a habitual place of stuffed-down anger.

I shocked my sister one day when my family was having dinner at a pizzeria. Our food had been served, and after a few bites, the waiter came over to ask the required, "And how is everything?" As Seinfeld captured beautifully in his famous episode "The Chinese Restaurant," no matter how bad things are, the habitual answer for most of us is a very enthusiastic, "Oh, very good, thanks."

But that day, I said, "Not good! Actually, I'm quite angry! I ordered whole wheat pizza, and this is not whole wheat!"

My sister stared at me with a look that said in equal parts, "You go, girl," and "*Psycho*..."

This went on for six weeks. I must say, people were very patient with me, especially my father; that man really loves me. Thanks, Dad — seriously.

Finally, I had paid my dues and done my work, and I was off the hook. As Luther told me in Princeton, "The mind is like a forest. To set up new pathways and habits requires bushwhacking." I had spent six weeks bushwhacking a new neural pathway in my brain. Now when I got angry, I knew it, and I could speak about it. My anger existed not as a vague, unidentifiable discomfort but as a clear, identifiable feeling. I now knew that I was mad, whom I was mad at, and why I was mad — right in the moment.

I went in for my next appointment with my teacher. He told me that the next step was to express the anger, not just in words, but, when appropriate, with emotion, by actually getting pissed. Not through my head, not just by speaking about it, but by feeling it in my body and showing it.

Some foot-stomping tantrums awaited me in my immediate future. In fact, I am a firm believer that if one skips a stage of development, he or she might actually have to relive that stage later on. So I was now unofficially four years old.

My teacher sent me away with the following homework:

1. Chant "o, oooh, ah," the vowel sounds of the base chakras, to build a sense of security and to connect with my body and emotions.

2. Chant "hahm," the mantra sound of the throat chakra, to open that channel and allow the anger to be expressed.

3. Lean a mattress against the wall in my apartment, and punch the mattress to release anger as part of my yoga practice every day.

I performed this homework sedulously. My yoga practice now consisted of warm-ups, postures, chanting, beating the shit out of the mattress, and then meditating.

The mattress made my knuckles bloody, so I had to wear my winter gloves. I'd chant while I boxed. Sometimes this turned into yelling, sometimes bawling. For some people, encouraging this sort of violence might be a terrible idea, but it was just what I needed. I connected to my power. I strengthened my base chakras. I opened my throat chakra. And in boxing the crap out of that mattress, I bushwhacked a channel for letting anger out of my body. It felt great.

The mattress took the brunt of my anger. It gave me a safe and healthy means of venting. In fact, while I might have stomped a foot once or maybe twice, and while I might have spoken quite firmly a few times, outside my mattress boxing matches, I was actually pretty relaxed and tantrum-free. My work in the six weeks of phase one, in learning to *recognize* the anger, had laid a strong foundation. Once I earnestly felt and mindfully acknowledged the truth of the anger, it could resolve pretty easily. It is really only blocked and repressed emotions that blow up and cause problems.

So over time I was able not only to feel when I was mad but also to express it and let it out. As I said, this practice did not turn me into a road-raging sociopath. Quite the opposite. When the channels are open, there is freedom of choice and swift resolution. When angered, I could feel my anger and *choose* whether or not it was appropriate to emote. Sometimes it's useful, sometimes it's not. Sometimes it's appropriate, sometimes it's not. Sometimes it's fair, sometimes it's not. And since my anger now was unobstructed, it would flow through me very quickly. Things that might seem huge if allowed to build up for hours, days, weeks, or years were like nothing when dealt with immediately. Something that after months of stewing might have required boxing a mattress till it drew blood from my knuckles now might require only a firm, "No thanks, I don't feel like pizza. Do you mind if we cook up some chicken tonight?" That's the thing. I was only angry because I had never advocated for myself. But now that I had bushwhacked a new path and felt free to speak up, I did not feel powerless, trapped, cornered, and resentful. My anger would pass in a flicker of expression.

Again, I think most anger is really our resentment at feeling powerless, trapped, and cornered. When speaking up for ourselves is an option, there's much less of a fiery charge and less to feel resentful about. Self-empowerment unblocks anger and prevents repression. It transforms it from a toxin that builds up into a passing energy.

And opening a channel for anger to flow, just as it had back in yoga teacher training in 1995, allowed me to be more present with all my emotions and with my heart, and once again I was bathed in love. I saw clearly that in living so much from my head, I had missed heartfelt connection. The head always has questions: "Am I enough?" "Why does she love me?" "Why do my friends like me?" "*Do* they like me?" The head can't really answer these questions because the answers are out of its domain. The head can only conspire to connect and can only think about connection.

The heart, in contrast, *experiences* the connection. And my Montclair anger experiment opened the door yet a bit wider for my heart to be heard and involved. I had moved to Montclair to gain experience in the business of running a yoga center. I had gotten that, yes, but I had also gotten a lot more.

This experience brought to mind Misha, from the Sivananda yoga ashram in California. He was mindful as he ate, mindful as he worked, and mindful as he played. He was ever committed to

God, chanting her name throughout the day. And most important, he faced every interaction and every moment with an open and full heart.

Misha's type of living has been an epiphany to me. I don't know if he was born with an open heart or if he had worked up to it. But I aspire to interact with the world, as Misha did, through my heart.

I find that if I open my heart before an interaction, I have a much more satisfying experience. One day recently, for example, I arrived home from work and my wife asked me to drive our sons' babysitter home. Our babysitter is twenty-five and very cool, and, more important, she loves my kids, which makes her flawless in my book. This was the first time I had spent any time with her (she's usually at the house when I'm at work), and I was afraid of saying the wrong thing, offending her, and losing our babysitter. This was absolutely ludicrous, and I knew that, since her relationship with my family is not so precarious as that, but for some reason it's how I felt in the moment.

After I dropped her off I felt sad. I realized that the whole time I had focused on what she thought of whatever I was saying rather than on truly connecting with her. I had missed an opportunity to share with a person who deeply loves my sons.

I am committed to opening my heart before every interaction. It takes a lot of work and a lot of reminding. But it's worth it. When I have lunch with friends, I can notice myself trying to be liked or entering a subtle contest to be the funniest or most interesting. It's exhausting. But when I'm Misha, coming from my heart, I relax, and our dynamic shifts to a few imperfect humans sharing and connecting. When I interact from my mind, I'm insecure and competitive, and ultimately alone. When I interact from my heart, I'm connected. That's the yoga that Misha taught me.

And here, then, thanks to that loving *meshugganah* Misha, we come to Key to Happiness number six:

**Connect with your heart,
and interact with others from that place.**

In other words, be Misha. It's much richer and more satisfying.

Recall Ram Dass's quote from the beginning of chapter 14. He said that there are three ways to be in the world — to be alone, to realize we are all connected, and to realize we are all one. The latter two are experienced through the heart and are a lot more fun.

Chapter 29

SLP

Yoga is the stilling of the mind
So that the yogi is centered in his heart.

— *YOGA SUTRAS*, lines 2–3

A few months later, in November, I was done with my work in Montclair, and I gave away my poor, beaten-up anger mattress, donated my sofa to the Salvation Army, stashed my boxes of pots and pans in my parents' basement, and headed to Kripalu for the Spiritual Lifestyle Program, a three-month residential volunteer program. I'd be washing dishes by day and training by night.

By now more men were attending Kripalu, so we were dispersed throughout the building, no longer confined to our one-room gypsy shantytown. Also, on a weekend visit to Kripalu a few months earlier, an anonymous roommate had ratted me out to the front desk as a snorer. This is a very serious accusation at Kripalu, and it caused me to get booted from the dorm and reassigned to a snorers' room.

I don't quite follow the logic on this one: "Hmm, this guy snores and is keeping everyone else awake. Let's put him in with other snorers...surely, they can't hear one another." Grouping snorers to protect nonsnorers seems cruel and unusual to me. If you prick us, do we not bleed? If you tickle us, do we not laugh? If you snore at us, do we not hear? I might as well have been chained to a radiator.

To be fair, I did notice that any time there was extra space in the building, the reservations department assigned each snorer to a separate room. This brought the epiphany, "Wait a minute, I get my *own* room?"

Suddenly the snoring black mark on my permanent Kripalu file didn't seem so bad. Several visits in a row, I humbly reminded the front desk of my snoring designation, was thanked for my honesty, and then enjoyed my single-room accommodations. This plan gave me several nights of quiet and solitude but proved to be quite myopic of me, because it turns out that the luxury snorers' accommodations were reserved for paying guests, such as I had been on those weekend visits. Snoring volunteers, like me now in the SLP program, on the other hand, were grouped together. And I was grouped with Cletus.

Cletus was many things. He was a real-deal hippy, straight out of the 1960s, and I think his laundry was from then too. He smelled of socks and patchouli, and he snored like a Mack truck.

The room Cletus and I shared was small, maybe seven feet wide. We each had a twin bed, and if you do the math, that puts our heads maybe four feet apart. On the first night it became clear that there was absolutely no chance of sleep. I picked up my blanket and wandered, Linus-like, through the building.

I settled into a couch in the common room and was awoken by security at 3:00 AM. Like a Central Park vagrant I was asked to move along. I told the guard of my plight, and she let me stay until morning.

In the morning I went to the front desk and begged to be mainstreamed into a men's dorm. I explained that eating dairy made me snore, and I vowed to cut it from my diet. Where else but in a holistic health center would the front desk clerk make a note of that in my file? I was provisionally allowed into room 115, with the warning that if anyone complained of snoring (or saw me eating yogurt in the dining hall), I'd be back in with Cletus. That was simply not an option for me, so I was resolute in my yogurt abstinence.

The first night in my new glorious mainstream dorm I was so afraid of uttering even a loud exhaling breath that I hardly slept. In the morning, exhausted and desperate, I accosted the others in the room, "I didn't snore, did I?"

"Who is this lunatic?" they must have thought.

In the end my dairy-free plan worked, and I spent the three months of SLP happily mainstreamed. In yoga classes, Cletus would often fall asleep during guided relaxation, and his porcine rumblings would burnish, buttress, and fortify my resolve against morning yogurt.

During the months that I lived and washed dishes at the ashram, I ate clean food, breathed fresh mountain air, and attended yoga classes and inspiring experiential workshops. I never felt healthier or more inspired. But the best part of my day at the ashram was the daily "share." At the end of our morning work shift, before lunch, we would meet in small groups and practice group colistening.

"Colistening" is Kripalu-speak for the practice of two or more people taking turns mindfully speaking and listening. The speaker reports sensations and feelings. The listener listens. Often the speaker and listener sit next to each other, even thigh to thigh, but facing in opposite directions. The goal is for the speaker to speak openly and honestly and for the listener to witness but not respond.

Group share was similar. We'd sit in a circle, with one person acting as the facilitator. The job of the facilitator was to move things along if one person monopolized the session, to bring people back to their own experiences if they got into a mindless rant about, say, how evil their supervisor was, and to remind listeners to only listen and witness.

The group is there to witness but not validate. Most people, when speaking eye-to-eye with someone, alter what they say based on their listener's gestures and facial expressions. This is not necessarily a bad thing, and it can be very valuable, like when selling encyclopedias or tutoring algebra, but the goal in this exercise is not to respond to others but to find and speak from one's *most real* inner experience.

The speaker reports her experience. Reporting can include physical sensations ("My lower back feels stiff"), thoughts ("My mind is spinning about what I'm going to do when I leave Kripalu next month"), or emotions ("I feel so angry at Tom for snapping at me about the trash this morning"). The goal is not to vent, which is *being lost in* the feelings, but to note sensations, thoughts, and feelings, which is *seeing/experiencing* the feelings. In this way, sharing is like assisted meditation.

I once heard a meditation teacher say that as he became more experienced in meditation, he would remember to snap out of his thoughts more often. So sharing is like cheating, like adding thirty years onto your meditation practice — allowing you to experience the state of being a seasoned, experienced meditator. When you are lost in thoughts, the facilitator snaps you out of it. She helps you shift from being lost *in* a feeling to *noting* and *experiencing* a feeling — being mindful of it. You become *most real*, identified with the deep, true you, rather than the passing thoughts.

∽

During my first month of the program at Kripalu I met Matt Oestreicher, and really he's the one who taught me how to share. As you know, if you've seen him perform as a musician, Matt has an uncanny ability to sense (and affect) the mood of his audience. Similarly, Matty can read a person's energy. He can see underlying motivations. He can see what a person is doing — not just what he thinks he's doing, but what's really going on.

So after our first group share together, Matty approached me and asked if he could relate an observation. Since most people only saw my facade of polished yogi, I welcomed his reflection. I expected, "You seem so at peace; you must have been meditating for many years."

But instead Matty said, "When you share, you lean forward. You're very invested in what people think about you. You're saying what you think will get them to respond rather than what you really feel."

When someone speaks directly to a person's core issue, one of two things can happen. Either the recipient is open and says, "Wow, you're right," and is ready to accept and change the pattern. *Or* the recipient is not open and says, "Fuck you very much, you assbag son of a bitch."

You might recognize this type of dynamic from when you last told your partner or friend that she was acting "exactly like her mother." She probably was. And she definitely did not like hearing it.

I'm sure you have experienced something like this yourself. Your spouse, parent, child, or best friend, someone who knows you ridiculously well inside and out, made an all-too-true observation that cut you to the core. You probably got very pissed. If a friend tells me that I'm not very creative, I think, "What a strange thing to say." I might be annoyed by the put-down, but I move on very easily, since deep down I know she's wrong. But if she says, "You're too heady today, you need more heart," I'm either in a receptive space and say, "Good catch, thanks," or I stew for three hours. And if I'm stewing for three hours it's because deep down, I know she's right, and it's the thing I like least about myself.

Matty, with his keen eye, had hit on a very sensitive point for me. He had actually seen me. The real me. And I knew he was right. I did speak too much to what I thought people wanted to hear. And I did spend *way* too much energy trying to be liked, trying to be funny, and trying to be attractive. I cared too much what others thought, and this kept me from experiencing my authentic self in relationships. I had done some good work experiencing my true self when alone in meditation — though even there I was always trying to impress the mental specters of my parents, my teachers, and every woman I had ever had a crush on. In interactions with others, I was a chameleon and a mirror for whom I imagined people wanted me to be.

So my response to Matty, at least in my own mind, was precisely, "Fuck you very much, you assbag son of a bitch!" But all that came out of my mouth was, "Huh."

I was pissed. I now hated this guy.

I hated Matty for a while. And then we became best friends.

But first, I stared him down from a distance. Then I sent him very angry, hard looks. And after a few days of hating on Matty from a distance, I decided to confront him. Damn that anger-releasing homeopathic! Remember, I had just completed my mattress-boxing-anti-anger-repression intensive in Montclair. (Notice, though, that I had actually regressed a bit and needed some time before I finally approached him.)

I told Matty that his observation had hurt my feelings and that I was angry.

Matty apologized, and I shared how very true his insight had been. That opened the door, and after that the friendship began.

Here was a major success of my anger project. A year earlier, I would not have confronted him. Not only would I have missed out on a soul brother, but also, in being so closed and guarded, I would have missed the opportunity to work on the very issue he had pointed out.

Matty was a kindred spirit, a fellow psychospiritual experimenter. Here's an example. A few weeks after we became friends, Matty was away from Kripalu, visiting his folks, and I bumped into his brother, Jeff. I asked Jeff what Matty was up to at home. Jeff replied, "Oh, you know, same as usual. He'll sit for two hours at the kitchen table, journaling about what he's experiencing as he takes each bite of his lunch."

Matty and I performed experiments together. We'd walk around town and follow the energy to see where it brought us. We'd pretend to be each other's parents and have conversations. We'd reenact painful elementary school memories to unearth and release stored hurt and repressed emotions. We'd have lunch in the Lenox Diner and try to speak only from our truest selves. Not from fear, not from conditioned patterns, but from a deep, authentic place. For me, this was our most important experiment. It birthed my process of seeking authenticity in all my interactions.

I was learning that being able to size people up and figure out how best to reach them had made me a great debater in high school and a successful teacher and tutor. But in personal relationships, it was keeping me from expressing my true thoughts and feelings.

As one of my Kripalu teachers said, "People want *you*, Brian, not a copy of themselves." About my girlfriend, Millie, he said, "Millie doesn't want a partner who shares every one of her beliefs; she wants someone who counters her sometimes, shows her new ideas sometimes, and makes her grow. Most important, she has chosen you and that's who she wants to hear from. Plus," he finished, "if in fact, she does not want the real you, then let's face it, you don't want to be in a relationship with her anyway."

He was right. And I practiced letting the real me show up in the daily share. It became my gymnasium. I'd practice speaking from the true Brian Leaf, not the Brian who said what people wanted to hear or made people laugh or made people like him.

I closed my eyes and spoke of what I actually cared about and what I actually felt. I could be happy, sad, angry, or apathetic. I closed my eyes to stay true to me, to avoid looking to the listeners for validation, to avoid adjusting my words in search of their approving nods and appreciative laughs.

I see now that this too has been a salient feature of my psychospiritual experiments these many years, from the Subway Coca-Cola cup I stashed under the seat in New Jersey to the Gymnasium of Sharing at Kripalu. I seek to have my personality reflect my true, deepest self. It's not that I need to be radically honest with everyone I interact with and to say everything on my mind. It's that I need to be radically honest with myself about what I'm thinking and feeling. I want to make choices from that place of transparent self-honesty, from the deepest, purest connection to my heart and soul.

Dr. Edward Bach taught that all disease results from a dissonance between the callings of our soul and the desires of our ego or personality. That's the purpose of his Bach Flower Remedies, to bring soul and personality into harmony. To make our personality a perfect representation of our soul. Then we are a clean vessel of perfectly flowing energy and vitality.

This authenticity could be *the* key. And it goes by many names. It is unconditional love — acknowledging and accepting the imperfect truth of reality, that which is *most real*. It is being present. "Be here now," as Ram Dass says.

And here is the link for me. Colitis, anxiety, ADD, repressing anger, and being *most real* are all connected. I was insecure and afraid of expressing my true self, so I did not. And then I resented all those who made choices for me. I repressed my resentment and other emotions too, so I experienced the world through the lens of my mind rather than through my heart and emotions. This left me unsure and ungrounded and even more insecure, creating an insecurity-repression loop. This was all very stressful. Physically, this stress and repression took a toll on my health and manifested as colitis. It was ungrounding and unsettling, so psychologically and behaviorally it showed up as anxiety and symptoms of ADD.

But being *most real* — speaking and acting from my true self, being present and authentic, and having unconditional love for reality — is exactly the opposite of all that. It is grounded, secure, calm, relaxed, peaceful, loving, and sweet. It is exactly the opposite of a state of repression, stress, colitis, anxiety, and ADD.

And so we find ourselves, dear friends, at our seventh Key to Happiness:

Speak and act from your true self.

You're doing yoga. You're following the ground rules, the *yamas* and *niyamas*. You're meditating and building concentration and mindfulness. You're opening your heart. Well, the heart is the doorway to the true self. It might even be one and the same. So now you are ready. It's time for your own psychospiritual experiment: Ask yourself throughout the day, "What am I feeling right now?"

Put it on your screen saver, above your bedroom door, and in your wallet. Silkscreen it on a shirt and spell it out with your Alphabits. Shout it from the rafters if you need to. And over time, with this query, you'll know what you really feel and who you really are. Eventually, you won't have to ask yourself the question — you'll be connected and already know in each moment.

This is what the world wants. It is your dharma, your destiny. You are here to bring you to the world. When you do that, you serve the world best, and you find the greatest satisfaction, peace, *and* happiness.

Chapter 30

Becoming Most Real

The highest achievement is seeing what is already there.

— AMRIT DESAI

In the Gymnasium of Sharing during the Kripalu Spiritual Lifestyle Program, I noticed how often I disapproved of and therefore tried to change my reality. For the previous decade I had been experimenting with how to eat (mindfully, healthfully), how to breathe (from my diaphragm rather than from my chest), how to sleep (without a TV on, in the dark) — basically how to live — so it made sense that I was sculpting my environment with care. I'd realize that staring too long at a computer before bed disturbed my sleep, so I'd rearrange my schedule to use a computer earlier. I'd realize that I wanted a living space that had close access to the woods, and so I'd move to have that.

But I also controlled what I thought. In meditation, I began to see that I was sculpting reality moment to moment — trying to re-imagine it. I noticed that at each moment, as reality showed itself, I was rejecting that reality and imagining a new and improved version.

For example, if I felt hurt, an uncomfortable feeling for me, I might convince myself that "Zach didn't mean to hurt my feelings, so I should just let it go." Worse, I might just repress and deny the feeling altogether: "I am NOT hurt... (*quick, think of something nice*: birds chirping, *Seinfeld*, Gwyneth Paltrow, Angelina Jolie, a shiny summer day at the beach)... Serenity now! SERENITY NOW!"

I wondered how it would feel, instead, to sit with the truth for a time rather than rejecting reality and calling for a more pleasant version. My mantra became "I live in Truth."

As I sat in meditation, whenever I noticed that I was disapproving of reality and trying to hatch up a new one, I would say, "I live in Truth," and just notice and sit with the truth of the actual reality that was already there.

At first this was very difficult, especially with thoughts and emotions — it was difficult to sustain my focus on an uncomfortable thought or feeling. So I took it down a notch and decided to use physical sensations, which would be easier to notice and stay with. I'd sit in meditation, and when I'd notice a slight discomfort in my body, perhaps in my neck, hip, or knee, rather than adjusting I'd just watch and allow and experience the discomfort.

My mind would, of course, sometimes wander, and I'd forget about what I was doing — watching and feeling a discomfort in my shoulder. But sometimes I could stay focused on the sensation for a long time and see it through, and that's when I split the atom. I found that when I stayed with a physical sensation long enough, eventually there would be a burst of energy. My body would flail up and then back as though from a chiropractic adjustment, the tension would release, and there'd be a delicious new comfort.

Eventually I could sustain my focus on an uncomfortable emotion as well. The emotion would take on an almost palpable feel with substance and texture, like a cloud. I could feel and nearly see it in or around my body. And as with physical sensations, when I could stay with it, there'd be a burst of energy, though the emotion bursts were actually larger than the physical sensation ones.

My original intent of this practice was to allow reality rather than deny it by imagining a new version. In allowing reality I was present. But over time, "I live in Truth" became "Wait for it, wait for it…" and I went from watching and accepting a sensation to staring it down, waiting for the burst.

I was no longer accepting reality as it unfolded; I was slyly rejecting reality by staring it down until it shifted. I was dominating rather than accepting and loving the moment. I did this for quite a while, and eventually I wound up pretty depressed.

The depression snuck up on me. Depression can be like that. Things just seem gray. When I finally noticed it, I didn't know why I was depressed. I suppose all along I had an idea that something in my model was off. But I was so excited about it, it seemed like a special gift, and the burst was so exciting. Finally, I put things together: I was depressed because I was denying reality by staring it down.

This was different from how I had previously ignored or re-imagined reality, but it was still a way of denying reality. Investment in the present, in reality, brings vitality, but denying reality disassociates and depletes and ultimately brings depression. So as I denied the present so many times every day, I was digging myself into a hole.

When I finally recognized this dynamic, I decided to bring some love into my meditation. Instead of staring reality down, I decided to love it as it was, to unconditionally accept the truth of my actual reality there and then.

I'd sit in meditation and notice a sensation and want to stare it down as I had for so long. But instead, I'd just hold it and notice it and allow it. I'd even notice and allow (although not pursue) my desire to stare it down. My mantra changed from "Wait for it…" to "I see you."

Not "I see you" in a threatening way like in a horror movie, but in the way the Best Buddies nonprofit organization uses it, "I see you; I acknowledge you; you matter to me." In fact, whereas "Wait for it" says, "You don't matter to me, and I can wait this out until you disappear," my new mantra, "I see you," says, "You matter, I love you."

After some practice, my new mantra gave me a burst, but a very different kind of burst. If the "staring it down" burst was pure white sugar, this one was warm baked apple — less unsettling and more nutritious. Rather than flailing with the burst, my muscles would soften, drop, and relax. I'd involuntarily sigh a sweet, contented sigh.

Imagine your favorite relative, maybe your grandma from when you were young, giving you a warm, soft embrace, stroking your hair, and sweetly saying, "I love you." That's how it felt.

I call this process *becoming most real*. My aim is to see not my imagined or desired reality — not the one I'm cooking up to soothe my discomforts and fears — but the reality that actually exists, the one that is *most real*.

One day I was meditating and feeling lethargic. I was asking, "What is *most real?*" and looking for the burst of energy. I was hungry for it, wanting to shift my sluggish state. I couldn't see anything beyond the low-energy daze I was in. I thought, maybe there is no most real right now, no high-energy state. And then, bang, it hit me. *"The low-energy state, my fleeing from it, and my search for a different, higher-energy state is*, in this moment, *most real."* With the realization, my muscles softened, my breath calmed, my mind relaxed, I smiled involuntarily, and I felt a renewed vitality.

Most real doesn't look a certain way. It is not shifting from one undesirable state to a different, more desirable one. It is only acknowledging and feeling whatever thoughts, emotions, and sensations are most true at any given moment. You acknowledge not the state you are trying to achieve but the state you are in. That is where true vitality lies.

Vitality comes not from a certain set of experiences but from simply acknowledging the truth of whatever is most real *right now.*

Yesterday I was stressed about a deadline for a few chapters I owed my agent. I was all worked up and feeling pretty miserable. I figured that if I could just stop feeling stressed and feel relaxed instead, then I'd be happy. So I breathed deeply, I meditated hard. I struggled. I pushed and fought — trying to talk myself out of it, trying to shift awareness, trying to trick myself, if necessary, into switching from feeling stressed to feeling relaxed.

But then I asked, "What is *most real?*"

I noticed that I was feeling tense and stressed. That I knew already. But I also noticed that I was struggling to change things, trying to force myself to feel relaxed. And that was the key. Because then I went from being lost in the struggle to being aware of the struggle. I went from identifying with the struggling to identifying with my deeper self that sees the struggle. For a moment I was grounded in the unflickering flame of my true self. For a moment I achieved the very aim of yoga and touched God.

In struggling to feel relaxed, I am rejecting how I actually feel. I am turning my back on reality and trying to cook up a new one. And this turning my back on reality denies the energy, the vitality, that is available in reality. In noticing, however, that I am feeling stressed *and* that I am struggling to feel differently, I acknowledge and experience that which is *most real.*

If I can find *most real* for even a moment in my morning meditation, or if during my day I am present for a few seconds with my struggle to shift reality, the struggle dissolves, and I am connected to my true self. I feel happier, more energetic, and more loving for the rest of the day.

⁓

All this has me wondering if my *shaktipat* experience with Genevieve back at Kripalu was not, in fact, botched, but rather precisely what I needed. The massive burst of energy that traveled up my spine and stopped at my heart may have been directed there in the first place. It was like a defibrillator, delivering a massive charge to my heart that began the process of its awakening. My heart had always functioned perfectly on the ordinary physical plane, but at a subtler level it was asleep, and I had been in cardiac arrest.

Living with what is *most real* is an awakening of the heart and of unconditional love. Conditional love says, "I accept reality if it looks like this," but true love from an open heart says, "I accept reality as it is, no matter what."

And this awakening of the heart is the same process that began to heal my ADD. When I can be *most real*, present to reality, grounded in my heart, in the truth of my being, I am unshakable, the opposite of spacey, distractible, and inconsistent. For many years, to balance my *vata* and calm my ADD, I did only one thing at a time, and I gave it my full attention. When brushing my teeth, I would just brush. When peeing, I would just pee. I was Daniel-son in the original *Karate Kid*. And this, at the time, served me well.

But I am now the father of two small children and am happy when I get to focus on only four things at once, such as brushing my teeth; helping Noah remember the words to the third, more arcane, verse of "Hot Cross Buns"; supporting little Benjamin as he climbs the toilet to flush; and wrestling with my old bacteriaphobic thoughts as Benjamin, in scaling the toilet, palms the vile, hairy space between the seat and the tank.

And all that is okay. My decade of training has prepared me for this. When I am *most real*, I can stay grounded, even amid the loving chaos. Now I can actually multitask. I just need to be mindful of whatever is *actually* going on in the moment, be it one, two, or twelve things, of whatever is *most real*.

This has been a continual epiphany for me: vitality comes not from trying to feel or act in a certain way but from acknowledging the truth of reality as it actually is in any given moment. When I am mindful of whatever is *really* going on in a moment, be it my mind wandering or being totally focused, it grounds me and fills me with energy. This practice shifts me from identifying with the ungroundedness to witnessing it and therefore identifying instead with a deeper, more centered me. Then the ungroundedness is a passing storm, and I remain calm and intact as it passes through.

So it turns out that my ADD — and I think this is true for everyone, whether or not they have been diagnosed with ADD — was not caused by my proclivity to be scattered and distracted. Those were the symptoms. I was scattered and distracted because I was not authentically grounded in the unflickering core of me. How scattering and ungrounding is it to try to be someone else, to try to have different thoughts and feelings? Conversely, when I acknowledge, accept, and then rest in my core, in my true self, I am grounded and present, and there can be no ADD. And this, again, is the wisdom of Kripalu yoga, and of yoga in general: to unite and integrate the private, internal self with the exterior self that interacts with the world. To be the same inside and out. To be grounded in the truest part of oneself and to let that part blossom into the world.

So here, at last, we come to Key to Happiness number eight:

Become most real.

This key is the meat of this book and the center of your charge. I often think of the scene in *Return of the Jedi* when Luke is fighting the emperor and at the same time Han and Lando are battling the empire's ships in space. These battles are happening simultaneously, and they both matter, but Luke's struggle with the emperor is what *really* matters. If he loses it, all fails. If he wins, game over. It's the same here. Doing yoga, following Ayurvedic guidelines, cultivating your intuition: these are all very powerful. But ultimately they are Han and Lando diddling around in the Millennium Falcon. Becoming *most real*, on the other hand, well, now you've awoken the spirit of Anakin Skywalker that still lives deep within Darth Vader, and you've transmuted darkness into the light.

You can practice this right now. Just ask yourself, "What is *most real*? What am I trying to feel right now, and what am I actually feeling right now?" These last two are related: What you are trying to feel right now, or, more specifically, the fact that you are trying, is what you are actually doing; it is *most real*. Again, *most real* is not the state you are trying to achieve but the state you are in.

And remember that what was *most real* ten seconds ago may not be *most real* now, so you have to stay in the moment with this. You must constantly inquire, "What is *most real*?" reaching into your body's sensations and into your emotions, noticing what is happening right now, mentally, physically, and emotionally, with each new moment.

Let's try this right now:

Notice the physical sensations in your body. Notice the feeling of your feet in your shoes. Feel your pants resting against your skin. Feel your shirt on your back. Notice areas of stiffness and areas of comfort in your body.

Then ask yourself, "What is most real?" This question can be expressed as words in your mind, or a wordless inquiry of feeling yourself more deeply. Notice if you have been struggling to ignore or change an aspect of reality. Notice if you have been fleeing a thought or sensation. Maybe your lower back is tight, and you're wishing it felt more relaxed. Maybe you feel great and don't want to lose the high. Maybe you're angry and feel like yelling. No problem. Notice and allow all of that for now. Simply notice that you are feeling these things. Notice whatever you are doing or feeling, and that you are doing or feeling it.

Any time you become lost in thought, come back to feeling your body and ask yourself, "What is *most real?*"

Practice for a few minutes.

Chapter 31

What Now?

Toward the end of my SLP stay at Kripalu, one day in the men's locker room, I found myself face-to-face with a naked Bikram Choudhury, self-proclaimed "yogi to the stars" and founder of Bikram yoga.

Bikram yoga is hot yoga: that means it is practiced in a room heated to 105 degrees Fahrenheit. The heat allows the muscles to relax and helps prevent injury. Bikram Choudhury was yoga champion of India four years running, and his yoga reflects that physicality and vigorousness.

I recognized Bikram and said an innocent, two-naked-men-in-the-locker-room "Hello." I think he was unaccustomed to my nonchalance — he truly is a very famous yogi, having taught the likes of Richard Nixon, Bill Clinton, Shirley MacLaine, Michael Jackson, Madonna, Lady Gaga, Indira Gandhi, and apparently Pope Paul VI. So after a few moments of chatting about the weather, he asked me, "Do you know the names of any famous yogis?"

I knew just where he was headed, and I'm not sure why I was so impish, but I named everyone I could think of — "Iyengar, Swami

Sivananda, Baron Baptiste, Amrit Desai" — but made no mention of him. So he asked, "How about Bikram Choudhury?"

He seemed to be having a good time with this. He was charged not so much with ego as with playfulness. Finally, I relented. "Yes, that's you." He was delighted at our game, and smiled the kind of winning smile you find on the faces of successful politicians and charismatic leaders.

"You should come to my workshop, for free, as my guest," he invited.

I would have liked that, I think, but I had to return to my afternoon shift washing dishes in the kitchen.

Like my disillusioning experience with Oskar years earlier, my interaction with Bikram opened my eyes. Before I met him, I had a pretty negative idea of what he'd be like. I imagined that he and his type of yoga would be plagued by competition and egotism.

And while he did, in fact, have a perfect, full-body tan and exactly the kind of toned frame you'd expect from a fifty-five-year-old ex-world-champion yogi, and while he definitely did seem to have a strong ego, that was not at all the whole picture. He was also charismatic, kindly, warm, and very vital. Additionally, he was playful, funny, generous, and open.

His intense hot yoga is not right for me, but it is probably perfect for someone of a different constitution. Maybe people who do Bikram yoga are not actually self-hating, self-flagellating masochists as I had imagined but are doing something very healthy and transformational for their body and soul. That's the whole point of Ayurveda, after all. We are all different, and different therapies, like different styles of yoga, are appropriate for different people.

When my three months of SLP were over, I extended for two months of assisting programs at Kripalu, and then I had to decide whether to stay on for six months of Karma yoga, the extended volunteer program. I sat for facilitation sessions with the director, I meditated, and I asked for inspiration.

It became clear to me that staying at this highly charged spiritual center, which would ordinarily be the fast road to growth, was actually not what I now needed most. Working in the world was my current charge. It was time. I had been moving around, studying, practicing intensively, and living in and out of retreat centers for a decade. Now I was ready to show up consistently for a relationship. I was ready to earn a living. I was ready to stay in one place and put down some roots.

Epilogue

Most Real

That the powerful play goes on,
and you may contribute a verse.

— WALT WHITMAN (and ROBIN WILLIAMS in *Dead Poets Society*)

*M*y path in holistic health had started in 1988 when I came down with ulcerative colitis. Through yoga and changing my lifestyle, I had healed the colitis. Through learning to feel and express anger, I had released my angst and opened my heart. Through Ayurveda, I had learned to keep my *vata dosha* in check, so I did not present with ADD anymore. I had learned how to eat, sleep, breathe, poop, emote, and love. And now I was ready to reenter the mainstream, but on my terms: living from my heart, following my intuition, seeking my bliss, being *most real*.

Joseph Campbell said, "Follow your bliss and the universe will open doors where there were only walls." I had been in a string of failed relationships with women whom I did not want to commit to, who were not truly available, or who did not want to commit to me, all of which felt safe to me. I had not really been ready.

But now I was expressing my true self, following my intuition, and following my bliss, and a door opened. Shortly after I moved from Kripalu back to Northampton, I met Gwen. We were engaged three months later. Several friends have described a similar experience.

Once they clarified their mission and committed to their true path, once they allowed their authentic self to come forward, their partner showed up.

✐

I was now certified as a yoga teacher, Ayurvedic practitioner, massage therapist, and holistic health educator. And I was soon to be certified in Reiki, craniosacral therapy, and Bach Flower Remedies. I decided to put this all to use by opening a stress-management practice in the nearby city of Springfield, Massachusetts.

I surveyed Springfield and arranged to teach a daily lunchtime stress-management class in a room rented at a church. I also made arrangements to use the room for private sessions. Plus, I figured I'd offer stress-management and wellness classes on-site in corporations. I could do one-time workshops or ongoing weekly classes.

I printed advertisements and business cards and went door-to-door. I spoke with employee assistance directors, corporate gym managers, and folks in human resources. I distributed pamphlets and met businesspeople eating in food courts and sitting in parks.

But being from the suburbs of New York City, I always make the mistake of thinking that every city will be like New York. And while Springfield may be the closest large city to Northampton, it is a city like New York in the way that a tofurkey is a turkey. This was not a bustling metropolis.

My intuition told me this was not to be, and I felt no bliss. There was no sense of rightness, and definitely no passion. So I abandoned my corporate stress-management plans.

Instead, I subletted space from a massage therapist right in Northampton. I called my practice Prana Bodywork Therapy, with the tagline "Come from your true self." I printed pamphlets and cards and sent out a mailing. I arranged to teach an eight-week holistic health class at a local yoga center, and I offered a free introductory evening to enlist students. I figured the series would feed clients to my private practice.

I designed my practice after the sessions my teacher gave me. I began each session by chanting, then we'd do yoga, massage, or energy work, and I'd prescribe Ayurvedic lifestyle suggestions or give a flower essence remedy to take home.

After a few months, however, I noticed that my energy work practice was not thriving. The only client who stuck with me was Litza, an eighty-seven-year-old woman whom I met while teaching a yoga class to Jewish seniors at the Holyoke Jewish Center. (These ladies ate me up. Every one of them had a granddaughter or grand-niece they were sure I should have married.)

What I did seemed funny to Litza, and in one meeting she admitted that she came for sessions only because I was such a nice Jewish boy and because I looked so much like her deceased son, Moishe.

Litza died a few months later, and her daughter called to thank me for my time with her. She said that in the final months of her life, Litza had found a lot of solace in our sessions and in "spending time with Moishe."

With my only client dead, I reevaluated my situation.

I urgently needed some cash flow. So I put up a few tutoring flyers. Almost immediately I received calls, and within a month, my tutoring business was thriving. I was soon booked.

A friend of mine back at the Holistic Health Association in Princeton kept a sign on her desk that read "What is trying to happen here?" I wondered that very thing. Why was my Prana Bodywork business flat but tutoring taking off? I wanted desperately to be a holistic practitioner, not a tutor. But I knew I needed to follow the energy of fate, and it had clearly spoken.

I was basically sixteen again, studying for the SAT, writing research papers, and filling out college applications, but now I was doing it with my students. At first, when kids got stressed or when we had too much to complete in one session, I'd get overwhelmed and my stomach would hurt. When parents would push, I'd invest too much in pleasing them and lose my center. I was the straight-A student, champion debater, and president of the Spanish Club all over again.

I was Bill Murray in *Groundhog Day*, sentenced to relive this time of my life until I got it right. I had to slug it out in the tutoring trenches until, instead of getting an ulcer, I could give it my all, stay focused, keep my center, and live from my true self.

And once I surrendered to tutoring, I loved it. The work was charged with energy and healing for me. And my business thrived. Having listened to my intuition and the flow of energy, having been *most real*, acknowledging the truth of reality, with all its parts, even when it was not what my mind or ego wanted, put me in exactly the right place: the right place for my talents, the right place to serve others, and the right place to make money. I helped a lot of kids. Teachers, principals, therapists, parents, and other tutors sought my counsel. I was fully booked, with a two-year waitlist.

My success and renown led to a book deal, and I authored ten successful vocabulary workbooks and test-prep guides. These books have been featured in magazines and used as props in television shows. (If you know your *Degrassi*, you may remember when Declan gives one to Holly J. as a going-away present.)

Listening to my intuition brought abundance and also, of course, joy. I loved connecting with the students. I loved their vitality. I loved seeing them gain confidence and grow. I also loved my schedule, the job's autonomy, and its room for creativity. I loved it, in fact, for eight more years, until I was ready. Until I had completed that piece of work. Until the energy shifted and tugged me in a new direction. Until it was time for my next experiment, and my next step toward freedom.

As I've said, you can't plan where you'll find bliss and transformation; you can only follow the whispers as they call out to you.

Author's Note

All the events depicted in these pages actually happened. Well, except for Zach and I visiting the one-hundred-year-old fruit-cake mentioned in chapter 13. We never made it there; I just like the idea of a one-hundred-year-old fruitcake. At times I have tweaked the timeline to simplify the narrative, and I have altered many of the characters' names. Otherwise the Princeton police, right now, as you read this, would be dispatching a squad car for Joshua. I have also, of course, changed certain identifying details, so, for example, Sara wouldn't know it was her butt I was talking about in chapter 8. D'oh! Sorry.

Acknowledgments

Thanks to all the terrific people of New World Library: Jason Gardner for championing my book and for a fantastic edit, Kim Corbin and Munro Magruder for spreading the word, Tracy Cunningham and Nate Williams for the inspiring design, Mimi Kusch for her uncanny eye for detail, and Marc Allen and Shakti Gawain for starting it all.

Thanks to my mom and dad, Susan and Manny Leaf, who even while scratching their heads, worried sick by my bewildering experiments, stood by me and loved me fiercely always. A son could ask for nothing greater.

Thanks to Julie Leaf, Larry Leaf, Matthew Oestreicher, Matthew Andrews, Joshua Sitron, Michael Brooks, and Ian Curtis for helping me find and express so many of my ideas.

Thanks to Pam Weber-Leaf for great editing tips, and to David Rice and Ian Curtis for their assiduous proofreading.

And, finally, of course, thanks most of all to Gwen, Noah, and Benjamin for love, time, support, and inspiration. Additional bows and gratitude to Gwen. She is the ultimate partner and mother, and I am truly blessed to know and love her.

Appendix 1

Sample Yoga Practice

*H*ere's a short sample yoga practice. The sequence helps you relieve stress, get energized, and focus your mind. We all have the potential to release fear, trust ourselves, and live freely.

You can record yourself reading the following directions and then play them back as you practice, or if you can't say the word *buttocks* without giggling, you can download a recording of me guiding the practice at www.Misadventures-of-a-Yogi.com.

So now, find a comfortable spot and get yoga-ing.

1. Alternate Nostril Breathing

Sit in a chair or on the floor with a blanket or pillow underneath your bum. Close off your right nostril with your thumb, and inhale slowly through the left nostril. Then close off your left nostril with your ring finger, and exhale slowly through the right. Then inhale through right, switch fingers, and exhale through left. Repeat this for a few minutes. This breath balances the right and left hemispheres of your brain. You can practice it anytime, even in your chair at work. If you get a strange look from your colleagues, just explain that you are balancing your hemispheres.

2. Skull-Shining Breath

Exhale sharply out through your nose as if blowing out a candle (*with your nose*), and then let the inhale come in naturally. Repeat for ten breaths. Then take one deep, relaxed breath. Repeat the process two times. This clears your mind — and your sinuses.

3. Cat Lift and Round (also called Cat/Cow)

Begin on your hands and knees, so you look like a coffee table. Inhale as you look up, allowing your back to arch down, and then slowly exhale as you look down, rounding your back up. Repeat ten times. This practice gently warms up the spine and nervous system, and relaxes the upper back and shoulders.

4. Mountain

Stand with your feet shoulder-width apart and parallel to each other. Press the crown of your head up toward the ceiling — chin parallel to the ground. Beginning with your arms at your sides, inhale as you slowly raise your arms out to the sides and up overhead (as though flapping your wings), and exhale as you slowly lower them.

Repeat this four more times, slowly moving your arms up and down, coordinating your breath with the movement.

The next time your arms are overhead, hold them there. Press your feet into the ground. Press your crown up toward the ceiling — chin parallel to the floor. Press your fingertips up toward the ceiling, simultaneously relaxing your shoulders. And breathe slow, deep breaths. Stay in this posture for eight breaths.

As you hold the posture, notice where you are straining. See if you can relax. Your muscles are working to hold up your arms, but your face, feet, buttocks, and legs can be relaxed. Soften your facial muscles. Relax your belly. Relax your feet and your neck. Practice being focused and alert, giving your all to the task, yet being relaxed and soft.

Now slowly lower your arms as you exhale.

Close your eyes and tune in to how you feel. Where do you feel strain?

Allow your body to make any small stretches or movements to release stress and tension. Open your eyes.

5. Half Sun Salute

Stand with your feet together, arms at your sides. Inhale as you flap your arms up halfway, so you look like a big T.

Then exhale, bending your knees a bit, and slowly fold over, hinging at the waist, to touch your hands to the floor. Then, again, hinging at the waist, inhale as you come up halfway, sliding your hands up your legs. Then, exhale to fold back down.

Finally, inhale to come all the way back up to standing. This practice warms up your whole body and helps you connect to the rhythm of your breath.

6. Downward Dog

Begin on all fours, with your hands shoulder-width apart. Press firmly down through all parts of your hands, including your fingers, and reach your tailbone (buttocks) into the air. Your body should resemble an upside-down V. Keep your knees a bit bent and reach your bum way up. This pose invigorates your entire body and mind, while also relaxing your shoulders and upper back. Stay in this posture for three relaxed breaths. Then slowly lower down.

7. Fish Pose

Lie on your back on a carpet or mat. Place a rolled-up towel underneath your shoulder blades as you lie on the floor. Breathe six relaxed breaths. This pose opens and stretches your chest, shoulders, and neck.

Remove the towel, close your eyes, and feel any sensations. Allow your body to make any small stretches or movements to release stress and tension.

8. Relaxation Pose

Lie on your back. Take a few deep breaths, allowing each exhalation to be a long sigh. Allow your body to relax and to be supported by the floor. Relax as your thoughts pass through your mind. Do not engage with them, just witness.

(You can sample a few minutes of relaxing music here, probably not DMX.)

After a few minutes, begin to deepen the breath. (*pause*) Feel your belly and chest rise and fall with each breath. (*pause*) Wiggle your fingers and toes. Then gently roll to one side and come to a seated position.

Notice how you feel after this yoga series. Set the intention to take this feeling into your day, into your relationships, into your work, into your life. Set the intention to notice your muscles as you go about your day. Notice when muscles that need not be activated are tense, such as a fist clenching while you're driving in traffic, and allow those muscles to relax, unclench, and soften. Notice when muscles are stiff, and allow your body to make any small stretches or movements to release tension. This will reduce your stress, increase your vitality, and make you happier.

Appendix 2

Sun Salutation

During the past twenty years I have seen countless approaches to and variations of sun salutation, but still I find myself practicing the series as Oskar taught it to me in 1989. Below are his instructions, as I recall them twenty years later.

Stand at the front of your yoga space. *Inhale.*

Exhale as you bring your hands into prayer position (palms touching in front of your heart).

Inhale as you reach overhead and bend slightly backward by pressing your pelvis forward.

Exhale as you bend forward, hinging at the waist and bending knees slightly.

Continue *exhaling* as you bring your hands to the ground next to your feet.

Inhale as you reach your right foot way back into lunge posture. *Exhale.*

Inhale as you bring the left foot back to meet the right into plank posture.

Exhale as you drop your knees, chest, and chin to the floor.

Inhale as you slide your chest forward and straighten your arms into upward-facing dog posture.

Exhale as you raise your buttocks high into the air into downward dog posture.

Inhale.

Exhale your right leg forward into lunge posture.

Inhale.

Exhale your left leg forward into standing-forward bend.

Inhale your arms out to the side, and bending knees slightly, hinge at the waist while bringing your arms up overhead and coming into a slight back bend by pushing the pelvis slightly forward.

Exhale your hands into prayer position.

Repeat.

Appendix 3

Meditation

Running builds your endurance. Bench-pressing builds your pecs. Sit-ups tone your abs. Similarly, meditation builds your concentration "muscles" and strengthens your ability to stay focused on what is *most real*.

To establish a meditation practice, choose a spot as your meditation area. Over time you will associate the space itself with meditation, which will allow you to settle into each day's practice more easily. Set up a cushion or chair to sit on. You can even light a candle or burn some incense before you sit.

If you feel distracted at the beginning of a sit, it helps to begin with a few minutes of alternate nostril breathing. (See the instructions in appendix 1.)

CONCENTRATION MEDITATION

Practice this concentration meditation until you feel comfortable staying focused. Then move on to the *most real* meditation, which comes next.

Read the following instructions several times before practicing. You can also record yourself reading the directions and then play them back as you practice. Or you can download a recording of me guiding the practice at www.Misadventures-of-a-Yogi.com.

Sit in a comfortable position on your chair or cushion. You need not imitate a swami with your legs twisted together. Then close your eyes. Relax your face. Relax your body. Sit up straight, but stay relaxed.

Become aware of your breathing. Find a spot where you notice your breathing, either the rise and fall of your belly or the in and out of air through your nostrils. Bring your attention to this place. Now, count ten normal breaths. Unless you're already a Zen monk or a superhero, your mind will probably wander. That's okay. You'll start counting, "One, two, three" and then wander off and think about food, work, sleep, or sex. Whenever you notice that your mind has wandered, gently come back to counting the breath. Start over at one. If ever you make it to ten breaths, start over counting at one. Do this for five minutes every morning and every night.

Meditation, like weight training, takes work and repetition. If you do these exercises every day, you will build your ability to focus. As you feel this ability strengthening, try the *most real* meditation exercise.

MOST REAL MEDITATION

Sit comfortably on your chair or cushion. Close your eyes. Relax your face. Relax your body. Sit up straight, but stay relaxed.

Become aware of your breathing. Find a spot where you notice your breathing, either the rise and fall of your belly or the in and out of air through your nostrils. Bring your attention to this place and count ten normal breaths. Whenever you notice that your mind has wandered, gently come back to counting the breath, starting over at one. If you make it to ten breaths, start over counting at one. Do this for a few minutes until you settle into the practice.

Then open your awareness beyond your point of focus to all

bodily sensations. Feel your pants resting against you skin. Feel your shirt on your back. Notice areas of stiffness and areas of comfort in your body. If you feel relaxed and focused, open your awareness to feelings and emotions. Continue counting breaths. Observe your sensations, feelings, and emotions, and use the breath as an anchor to stay focused and present. If you notice that your attention has wandered, come back to the breath and to experiencing sensations and feelings.

Now ask yourself, "What is *most real?*" This question can be expressed as words in your mind, or as a wordless inquiry of feeling yourself more deeply. Notice if you have been struggling to ignore or change an aspect of reality. Notice if you have been fleeing a thought or sensation. All these are okay to do; simply notice that you are doing them.

Vitality rests not in the experience you think you need to have, but in the truth of your actual experience.

Any time you become lost in thought, come back to counting and feeling the breaths. Ask yourself, "What is *most real?*"

Practice for twenty minutes.

∽

Notice how you feel after practicing. Allow yourself to transition gently back to daily activities, and set the intention to bring the inquiry "What is *most real?*" into the rest of your day.

Appendix 4

Colistening

$\mathcal{S}$it side by side with your partner, facing in opposite directions. One person goes first and speaks, and the other person witnesses without validating or responding in any way. The speaker reports her experience. Reporting can include physical sensations ("My lower back feels stiff"), thoughts ("My mind is spinning about the presentation I gave at work today"), or emotions ("I feel so angry at Tom for snapping about the trash this morning"). The goal is not to vent (which is *being* the feelings), but to note sensations, thoughts, and feelings (which is *seeing/experiencing* the feelings).

The listener listens without validating. You can decide together if you will later be allowed to discuss things that came up. Sometimes it is more freeing to know that your partner will not try to solve any problems you discuss.

After some time, the speaker says, "Pass." Both partners pause, and then the listener becomes the speaker. You can each have one turn, or switch roles several times. You can keep the time periods flexible, or you can time each other. In that case, the listener times for, say, three minutes, and then says, "Time," when the allotted time period is over.

Appendix 5

Guided Relaxation

I f you read the following relaxation exercise as prose, it sounds kind of insane, or at least ridiculously dull. But that's the whole point. Record it into your iPod and have at it, and you'll see. Your stress will fall away, and your muscles will be mush in sixty seconds flat. (You can also download the sequence as a free podcast from my website: www.Misadventures-of-a-Yogi.com.)

Lie down on your back and close your eyes.

Take slow, deep breaths.

Bring your awareness to your feet. Allow your feet to relax, like a fist unclenching.

Bring your awareness to your calves and shins. Let these muscles relax and soften and unclench.

Bring your awareness to your thighs and hips. Allow the thighs and hips to relax and unclench.

Bring your awareness to your whole legs. Allow the legs to relax even more, to soften even more. Allow all the muscles to drop, allow yourself to be fully supported by the floor.

Now, bring your awareness to your pelvis. Allow your pelvis to relax, to unclench, and to drop and be supported by the floor.

Bring your awareness to your lower back. Allow your lower back to relax and drop.

Bring your awareness to your belly. Allow your belly to relax, to unclench, to let go.

Bring your awareness to your upper back and chest. Allow your upper back and chest to relax, to unclench.

Bring your awareness to your shoulders, arms, and hands. Allow your shoulders, arms, and hands to relax, to unclench, to soften.

Bring your awareness to your whole neck. Allow your neck to relax, to unclench, and to soften.

Bring your awareness to your face: eyes, nose, mouth, and cheeks. Allow your face to soften, to relax, to unclench.

Bring your awareness to your scalp. Allow your scalp to relax.

Now bring your attention to your whole body: feet, legs, pelvis, belly, back, chest, arms, neck, head. Allow all your muscles to relax even more, to unclench even more. Allow all your muscles to soften and drop even more, allowing your whole body to be supported by the floor.

Now relax for a few minutes.

(Let two minutes pass on the recording. You can sample relaxing music here, probably not AC/DC.)

Now gently begin to deepen the breath. Breathe slow, deep breaths.

Wiggle the fingers and toes.

Slowly roll over to your right side and open your eyes. Slowly sit up and set the intention to bring this feeling of relaxation and calm into your day.

Appendix 6

Ayurvedic Constitutional Survey

$\mathcal{F}$ ill out the following Ayurvedic constitutional questionnaire. For each row, circle characteristics in the one or two columns that best describe you for that trait.

	VATA	PITTA	KAPHA
BONE STRUCTURE	thin, slight	moderate	broad
BODY WEIGHT	difficult to gain	moderate	easy to gain
SKIN	dry, cool, dark	soft, oily, warm, fair	thick, oily, cool, pale
HAIR	black, dry, kinky	soft, oily, yellow, early gray, red	thick, oily, wavy
APPETITE	variable	strong	slow, but steady

Continued on next page

	VATA	PITTA	KAPHA
THIRST	variable	strong	low
MIND	active, restless	aggressive, sharp	calm, slow
EMOTIONAL TEMPERAMENT UNDER STRESS	fearful, insecure, unpredictable	aggressive, irritable	calm, greedy, attached
RESOLVE	changeable	fanatic	steady
MEMORY	recent good, long term poor	sharp	slow, but prolonged
DREAMS	fearful, movement	fire, anger, violence	watery, romantic
SLEEP	interrupted	little but sound	heavy, prolonged
SPEECH	fast	sharp, cutting	slow

Adapted from Vasant Lad, *Ayurveda: The Science of Self Healing: A Practical Guide* (Lotus Press, 1984).

The sum of the checks down each column indicates the number for *vata*, *pitta*, and *kapha*. If one of these numbers is much larger than each of the others, such as 11 *vata*, 4 *pitta*, and 3 *kapha*, then that *dosha* is the one to watch for imbalances.

You can also confirm your results with the following cheat sheet:

1. Under stress, I become _____.
   A. scattered and anxious
   B. focused and angry
   C. stuck

2. When I'm hungry, I get _____.
   A. scattered and anxious
   B. angry
   C. depressed

3. I hate to feel _____.
   A. too cold
   B. too hot
   C. too wet

4. My biggest psychological struggles involve _____.
   A. anxiety
   B. being judgmental, irritation, anger
   C. feeling stuck

5. When I have digestive problems, they involve _____.
   A. intestinal gas and bloating
   B. heartburn
   C. slow digestion, feeling stuck

6. When I get sick, I feel _____.
   A. Worried, fried, constipated.
   B. Fevers, skin rashes, diarrhea.
   C. Congested, stagnant, blocked up.

Count the number of As, Bs, and Cs. Mostly As indicates *vata*, mostly Bs *pitta*, and mostly Cs *kapha*.

Appendix 7

Ayurvedic Recommendations

*O*kay, now choose three or four of the following recommendations for your constitution, and apply them in your life. Do this for at least three weeks. Let us know how it goes at www.Misadventures-of-a-Yogi.com.

To balance *vata*:

1. Keep warm.
2. Give yourself soothing oil massages.
3. Eat mostly cooked foods and use a bit of spice.
4. Keep a regular routine, and look over your schedule at the beginning of each day, so your mind can relax and know what's coming.
5. Wear soft, comfortable clothing.
6. Practice gentle forms of exercise and yoga.
7. Spend quiet time in nature, ideally near a lake or gently flowing stream.
8. Avoid or cut back on caffeine, wheat, sugar, and processed foods.

To balance *pitta*:

1. Keep cool.
2. Get lots of fresh air, but avoid too much direct sun.
3. Eat lots of fresh fruits and vegetables.
4. Avoid very spicy, very salty, and very oily foods.
5. Express your feelings in constructive ways.
6. Take evening walks in the moonlight.
7. Avoid or cut back on caffeine, wheat, sugar, and processed foods.

To balance *kapha*:

1. Get lots of vigorous exercise, every day.
2. Avoid fatty and fried foods.
3. Eat lots of veggies and cook with a bit of spice.
4. Eat less bread.
5. Avoid getting in a rut. Try new things, take challenges, travel.
6. Encourage your creativity. Draw, paint, sculpt, sing, dance, play an instrument, imagine.
7. Practice expressing your voice and your feelings.
8. Avoid or dramatically cut back on wheat, sugar, and processed foods.

About the Author

Brian Leaf, MA, is the director of the New Leaf Learning Center, a holistic tutoring center in Massachusetts. In his work helping students manage ADD and overcome phobias concerning standardized tests and math, Brian draws upon twenty-one years of intensive study, practice, and teaching of yoga, meditation, and holistic health. He is certified by the New England Institute of Ayurvedic Medicine and holds licenses or certifications as a yoga teacher, massage therapist, energy worker, and holistic educator. He also incorporates Bach Flower Essences, craniosacral therapy, Reiki, shiatsu, and tai chi into his work.

Brian is the author of eleven books, including *Name That Movie!* and McGraw-Hill's *Top 50 Skills for a Top Score*. His books have been featured on the CW, MTV.com, Fox News, and Kripalu.org.

Brian lives in western Massachusetts with his wife and two sons. His website is www.Misadventures-of-a-Yogi.com.

NEW WORLD LIBRARY is dedicated to publishing books and other media that inspire and challenge us to improve the quality of our lives and the world.

We are a socially and environmentally aware company, and we strive to embody the ideals presented in our publications. We recognize that we have an ethical responsibility to our customers, our staff members, and our planet.

We serve our customers by creating the finest publications possible on personal growth, creativity, spirituality, wellness, and other areas of emerging importance. We serve New World Library employees with generous benefits, significant profit sharing, and constant encouragement to pursue their most expansive dreams.

As a member of the Green Press Initiative, we print an increasing number of books with soy-based ink on 100 percent postconsumer-waste recycled paper. Also, we power our offices with solar energy and contribute to nonprofit organizations working to make the world a better place for us all.

Our products are available
in bookstores everywhere.
For our catalog, please contact:

New World Library
14 Pamaron Way
Novato, California 94949

Phone: 415-884-2100 or 800-972-6657
Catalog requests: Ext. 50
Orders: Ext. 52
Fax: 415-884-2199
Email: escort@newworldlibrary.com

To subscribe to our electronic newsletter, visit
www.newworldlibrary.com